The Hologram

VAG ABO NDS

Series editor: Max Haiven

Also available

001
*Pandemonium: Proliferating Borders of
Capital and the Pandemic Swerve*
Angela Mitropoulos

002

The Hologram

Feminist, Peer-to-Peer Health for a Post-Pandemic Future

Cassie Thornton

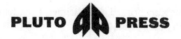

First published 2020 by Pluto Press
345 Archway Road, London N6 5AA

www.plutobooks.com

Copyright © Cassie Thornton 2020

The right of Cassie Thornton to be identified as the
author of this work has been asserted in accordance
with the Copyright, Designs and Patents Act 1988.

British Library Cataloguing in Publication Data
A catalogue record for this book is available from the
British Library

ISBN 978 0 7453 4332 7   Paperback
ISBN 978 0 7453 4333 4   PDF eBook
ISBN 978 0 7453 4324 2   Kindle eBook
ISBN 978 0 7453 4323 5   EPUB eBook

This book is printed on paper suitable for recycling
and made from fully managed and sustained forest
sources. Logging, pulping and manufacturing processes
are expected to conform to the environmental stand-
ards of the country of origin.

Typeset by Stanford DTP Services, Northampton,
England

Simultaneously printed in the United Kingdom and
United States of America

VĀG
ABO
NDS

Contents

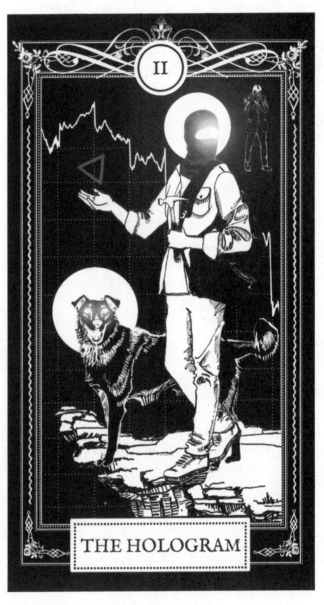

THE HOLOGRAM

Art by Amanda Priebe

The Fool

by Stella Lawless,
The Hologram's Resident Witch

The zero. The beginnings that tell us that, if we had any idea what we were getting into, we'd never do anything. Fools are dangerous as we know from past experience. And they speak truth to power when no one else can, *à la* the jesters. As for overcoming: whatever obstacles, stalls, walls or barriers you come across are there to make you stronger. We don't know what we don't know and we can't know it until we try. Fool cards are often people on a precipice about to take a step into the unknown. This is major, bigger than the ten of swords, which is a conclusion. The fool is always the beginning part of us. The part of us willing to do what's never been done before. Willing to wait for a train that might never come. Willing to walk forward in innocence and ignorance ... that part of us that's never been scorned or wounded or failed, that keeps going. It's that part of us that poet Wendell Berry writes about when saying "praise ignorance, for what man has not encountered he has not destroyed." This card has come up more times than I can count during the pandemic. Lots of swords too. This is the card of going and being and knowing there is no arriving. A loyal dog reminds us to bring allies with us on our journeys. The real treasure is in the beginning that is before the beginning. Look at the Hologram afresh and keep looking with love. You're walking the edges and it's impossible to know much more than that except that when it's time to go, you've got to.

VAG
ABO
NDS

Acknowledgments

"Feminist Economics and the People's Apocalypse" first appeared online in *GUTS Magazine* issue 8: Cash (15 June 2017).

"Art, Debt, Health and Care" first appeared on the website of Furtherfield Gallery and was printed in *State Machines: Reflections and Actions at the Edge of Digital Citizenship, Finance, and Art*, edited by Yiannis Colakides, Marc Garrett and Inte Gloerich (Amsterdam: Institute for Network Cultures, 2019). It has been updated.

A different version of "A Different Medicine is Possible: Visiting the Greek Solidarity Clinics" first appeared in *For Health Autonomy: Horizons of Care Beyond Austerity—Reflections from Greece,* edited by the Carenotes Collective (Brooklyn: Common Notions, 2020).

A different version of "Wikipedia Entry from the Future" was commissioned by *Arts of the Working Class* and will be distributed at the Venice Biennial in 2020, if it happens.

VAG
ABO
NDS

Foreword

Max Haiven
Series editor

The Hologram is something between an interventionist art project, a collectively improvised science-fiction story and a form of social activism directed at the way we reproduce ourselves and our social life together. At its simplest it is a protocol whereby three people (a triangle) can gather, online or in person, to provide intentional care, attention and support to a fourth person (the hologram). Its deceptive simplicity is a delivery vehicle for a radical vision of a different world, teaching its participants to become post-capitalist animals and helping them grow the strength, skills and solidarity for the revolutionary struggles Cassie Thornton hopes will soon transform the world.

Around 2015 one of Cassie's oldest friends called her a "brilliant healer" in a kind and supportive email. I've never seen her so vexed. By this time Cassie had begun to tire of hypnotizing people to get them to talk about debt, a practice she had begun as a heavily indebted MFA student in California and an activist with the Occupy Wall Street off-shoot Strike Debt. This was part of an approach to social practice or participatory art that had brought her some notoriety, especially in the San Francisco Bay Area where she was trying to live, less and less successfully as the tech bros human resources of Google, Apple and Facebook made the city into their stupid playground.

Cassie, who grew up in the working-class exurbs of Chicago to a family that struggled profoundly with debt, has a deep and abiding allergy (maybe even hatred) to the middle-class saccharine, self-congratulatory, individualistic, crypto-masochist, quasi-activist rhetorics of healing, self-care, pleasure, generosity and kindness. But, being a Scorpio, she cannot resist destroying them from the inside. Partly as Bay Area survival-strategy, partly as vengeance, she trained to become a Kundalini yoga instructor and began teaching Feminist Economics Yoga, reasoning that it offered her unparalleled access to the vulnerable unconsciouses of the personnel of the corporations she wished to annihilate. In other words, she thought of it as a form of anti-capitalist sabotage in an age when capitalism is deeply invested in the subjectivity of its workers.

As the reader will discover, a visit to crisis-ravaged Greece in January 2016 gave the impetus to *The Hologram* when Cassie met and interviewed many protagonists in the Greek solidarity clinic movement. As austerity decimated the nation's health care system and worsened broader indicators of health (poverty, social discord, hopelessness), groups of volunteers and healthcare practitioners came together not only to provide free forms of care, but to reinvent what health care might be in a more holistic, egalitarian and non-hierarchical way. Back in the United States one of Cassie's closest family members had recently died prematurely deeply in debt because they lacked access to affordable health care. She began to develop a plan to bring the idea of *The Hologram* home, as revenge.

At this time, Cassie was also working with a set of friends, all of whom were women struggling to survive as artists and activists in gentrifying cities, to workshop ways to provide support to one another amidst lives lived in constant flux and precarity. They were attempting to form an Intentional Community in Exile and *The Hologram* eventually emerged as one "social technology" from these discussions and experiments. It was refined as part of a series of four exhibitions titled *Sick Time, Sleepy Time, Crip Time: Against Capitalism's Temporal Bullying*, curated by Taraneh Fazeli in New York (Elizabeth Foundation for the Arts), St. Louis (The Luminary), Omaha (Bemis Centre) and Detroit (Red Bull Projects).

In the exhibitions themselves, Cassie presented a series of sculptural pieces of "collective psychic architecture" largely made out of the infrastructure of the gallery itself (old plinths, plexiglass donation boxes, broken chairs). These sought to reveal the forms of "bad support" that art institutions typically provide for artists, especially sick and disabled artists: "support" that promises to help you thrive when it actually extracts your labor, time, and care.

But behind the Bad Support project of institutional critique, *The Hologram* was growing. With Taraneh's care and help, Cassie began a series of practical experiments, piloting the basic model of the Hologram, where three people direct their intention and interest toward the well-being of a fourth. Dragooning gallery staff and artists into participating, *The Hologram* spored like a fungus among women and femmes in the dank, precarious and exhausted back rooms of the art world, among those who had been made into its infrastructure. To explore and workshop the ideas for *The Hologram*, Cassie taught Feminist Economics Yoga in community venues attached to the exhibition.

In 2019, Cassie began a collaboration with Furtherfield Gallery in London, initiated through an interview about *The Hologram* with its co-founder and co-director Marc Garrett, which is reproduced in slightly edited form in this book. Since then, Cassie has worked closely with Ruth Catlow (the gallery's other co-founder and co-director) on advancing *The Hologram* as a very unique interventionist artwork.

Furtherfield's status as the England's oldest institution dedicated to the intersection of art, digital technologies, and social change proved to be of tremendous importance when, almost as soon as Cassie arrived to take up a residency at the gallery in February 2020, the world was hit by the (at the time of this writing ongoing) Covid-19 pandemic. With Furtherfield's help, Cassie pivoted *The Hologram* project online. This has so far included a public workshop to introduce people to the ideas and practices of *The Hologram*, a four-part intensive course (reflected in this book) that trains enrollees to "become" future Hologram participants, and the piloting of a "Minimum Viable Hologram" program, which will pay participants to do one-time or short-term experiments with the *The Hologram's* protocols.

This book, then, presents materials and background to *The Hologram* as a work in progress. Yet the work of *The Hologram* will never be "done," even if Cassie herself moves on to other projects. Fundamentally, *The Hologram* is a kind of virus. One of Cassie's deepest inspirations has been Melanie Gilligan's fascinating 2010 film *Popular Unrest*, in which an increasingly digitally integrated form of capitalism, which controls nearly every aspect of life, accidentally produces a counter-tendency: "groupings" of individuals mysteriously brought together by a sense of irresistible solidarity. Cassie's dream, explored in "Wikipedia Entry from the Future," is that *The Hologram* becomes a kind of viral protocol that takes on a life of its own, a kind of lightweight, alternative model for revolutionary social reproduction.

I must disclose that I am no neutral or disinterested party: near the time when Cassie began the work that would become *The Hologram* we became partners in life and crime. I have therefore had a backstage pass to its whole fraught development. But it is for that reason I am so thrilled to hope that, through this volume, it might continue to reach an ever broader audience and embrace its promise to become a new habit of life for those of us who know a better world is possible.

VĀG
ABO
NDS

Preface: Artist's Update

I'm an artist and the current steward for *The Hologram*. One day it will live on as an autonomous, leaderless, everyday practice through the people who use it. For now, I'll be your tour guide.

My name is Cassie and I am an artist. That is partially why *The Hologram* is identified as art rather than a health project or a social science project. An artist is what they sometimes call you, if you're lucky, when you insist on surviving without a capitalist job. In another, non-capitalist time, and in a time that might yet come, I may have a more central role: problem solver, wizard, professional emoter. I believe that art should be democratized and the art world in all its preciousness should be abolished. But for now I use my role as an artist to do things that surprise people. I call it art to move these projects outside of our world of bureaucracy, regulation and skepticism. I do most of this art without money. I use art to make interventions because calling it art somehow allows people to be surprised, awed and open in ways they would not otherwise be. For many years I have worked as an artist, sometimes under the banner of the The Feminist Economics Department (me and occasional accomplices) to make "art" about and against what capitalism does to our imagination.

A lot of that work is tied to activism, for instance against debt, the focus of my work for many years. Recently I've became more and more interested in collective debts and their impact on the physical, mental and social health of individuals and collectives. That's what brought me to *The Hologram*.

After a year of planning, I arrived in London on March 2, 2020 to begin a three-month art residency at an arts organization called Furtherfield to do research and outreach that could grow *The Hologram*. Because *The Hologram* is an extremely challenging social project (one that highlights many of my greatest insecurities), I had avoided it while obsessing over it for years. I was not sure if I had the social skills and strategies necessary to deliver it to the world. I was also not sure what world would want or need it.

In early March, during the only in-person event of the residency, 25 people gathered around big tables at Furtherfield's Commons, a small space located in the city's Finsbury Park. There was hand sanitizer on the tables (which went unused) like socially necessary decor, and in those days we were still hugging, even strangers. In the second half of the workshop we did a visualization paired with some breathwork and movement. We breathed heavily with our mouths open as we moved our arms. We sweat and spluttered all over each other. We imagined going through a wall made of our collective anxiety, betrayal and disappointment, one that kept us from seeing our shared potential to cocreate the systems of care and community we need to thrive. Many people in the group imagined getting stuck in the wall rather than making it to the other side. One participant described the UK's universal and free National Health Service (NHS) as "the pinnacle of civilization." As a US citizen, I did not understand what she was talking about.

A week later, as the Covid-19 pandemic broke, I realized that I would not be leaving London, nor my apartment, for a long while. As people all over the world went into lockdown, I felt as if I had been placed inside of a dream locked in a nightmare. I felt that, suddenly, all the things that I had been screaming into the wind as an activist and artist had become common knowledge. It had become apparent to most people that many of the systems that had been pretending to care for us were only interested in profit. In some cases, it was that the systems had been so hollowed-out by cuts and bureaucratization they couldn't help but fail when we needed them most. In the pandemic, care and support became more valuable than money. People began discussing new ideas for how to organize care for others who could not leave their homes. At the same time, this potential was caught up in fear, mourning and death as systems we had been told to rely on failed us.

The central thesis of *The Hologram* is that all our crises are connected and that we are all a little sick. The pandemic revealed how remarkably connected we are, even when many of us live in relative isolation inside a hyper-individualistic culture. Ideas went viral in the pandemic as we learned how quickly something invisible (besides finance) can grow and connect us, how entangled all humans are (across national boundaries), and how quickly things can change (or how fast huge structures can crumble). If Covid-19 hadn't destroyed so many of our beliefs in the false systems of care and governance, I don't know if so many people would have so voraciously sought new solutions to what is now called "the crisis of care." I don't want to seem like an opportunist, but it is only because of the rupture in life created by the virus that something as weird as *The Hologram* could be seen as possible, or useful.

It is my sincere hope that this book becomes useful to you, in lockdown or after. Even though I am hiding behind or between these words, I am still just a person on a couch. You can easily find me here. Feel free to give me a call: I would love to personally welcome you to *The Hologram*.

Note on Terminology

The Hologram refers to the project as a whole, whereas "a Hologram" (capitalized but not italicized) names a group of four people, made up of a person, "the hologram" (not capitalized) who receives the care of a "triangle" of three people. This wording is intentionally ambiguous as it aims to sensitize us to the fluid boundaries between us.

VĀG
ABO
NDS

A Different Medicine is Possible: Greek Social Solidarity Clinics

On my way to visit the Social Solidarity Health Center (SHC) of Thessaloniki, Greece's second largest city, in the winter of 2017, I passed by a woman who was selling rings on the main commercial street. Andromeda had made each ring by hand. I picked one out with an old drachma, the pre-euro Greek currency, set like a gem. Most of the rings were made using a copper wire, coiled to capture and hold whatever kind of focal object she selected. Often, small scraps of leather and sometimes gems were entangled in a mess of wires that happened to also cling onto one's finger.

Andromeda was an unemployed microbiologist. She liked using copper because of its metallic property to sterilize what it touches. She told me that simply wearing a copper ring would sterilize the hand up to 99 percent, an overstatement. I told her I was walking back from the Solidarity Clinic, and she knew where it was, though she had never visited. The next day I read an article "'Patients Who Should Live Are Dying': Greece's Public Health Meltdown," which focused on the spread of preventable disease and a lack of care due to cuts amounting to about a third of Greece's total public healthcare budget.[1] Diseases were said to spread in part because overworked doctors didn't have time to wash their hands and patients were being put in dirty hospital beds.

Debt: Bringing the World Together in Crisis

In January 2017 I visited several solidarity clinics in Greece that served not only Greeks, who have been abandoned and punished by international debt markets, but also refugees, who have become trapped in the country thanks to the closing of Europe's borders to them. The solidarity clinic movement rose to prominence during the anti-austerity "indignados" uprisings of 2010 and 2011.

These clinics have become shining examples of mutual aid in crisis. Established in unused storefronts, offices or apartments—often squatted—they are staffed by medical professionals (doctors, nurses, technicians, dentists and more) who volunteer their time or come out of retirement, but also by non-professionals who serve in administrative and clinical roles. The clinics challenge typical medical hierarchies and bureaucracies, operated not by executives and administrators but by regular assemblies of volunteers, users of health services and members of the community. While they can only offer limited primary-care services they maintain relationships with health professionals in the mainstream medical system to ensure they can refer those in need to more specialized procedures, tests and care.

At that time, living in the United States, the idea didn't tempt my imagination because it was so far from what I could imagine wanting. As a white US citizen, even one without health insurance, I assumed that I would never need to stoop down to accept or desire free, community-run health-care. I pridefully absorbed the idea that good health care was expensive, even if it excluded me. After spending years researching and organizing around *personal* debt and its effect on collective and individual psychological, behavioral, social and emotional life, I began to become curious about the ways that *public* debts, like the one that encumbered Greece, work and how people internalize and live with those debts.

Until Trump's election, many US citizens lived as if everything was ok, even if it wasn't. That has now changed. Our culture bases dignity on our ability to pay for services. It's a culture that created Trump and that also created each of us, and one that loads regular people with so much debt (for housing, healthcare, education, transportation and public services) that it breeds numbness, obedience, isolation and narcissism. The hyper-individualistic character created by the debt keeps us from the sort of radical problem-solving that emerges in states of emergency, as it has in Greece. Greece's crisis is not only "theirs" but also "ours," though we may not know it yet. It is the crisis of global capitalism that puts its own reproduction ahead of ours.

Hearing Greek people tell me about the personal effects of the financial crisis was complex and terrible. But in a strange way, several people I

3

talked to told me the crisis came as a relief. I met a group of middle-aged women who cited "the crisis" as the birth of their new lives as radicalized people within activist communities, people who had found a purpose, who were now more than just workers and consumers. They felt powerful, connected and interdependent for the first time. To them, there have always been problems, but after they witnessed massive unemployment, huge taxes, home foreclosures and cuts to all public services they were forced to deal with what was earlier hidden. As American anthropologist Heath Cabot explains, the "second face" of the crisis is solidarity.[2]

Free (as in Freedom) Care (as in Interdependence)

In Thessaloniki, the early days of the crisis which saw the emergence of grassroots solidarity clinics also saw a radical worker takeover of an owner-abandoned tile factory called VIO.ME.[3] The Solidarity Health Center responded positively to the suggestion by the VIO.ME workers to create a health center there. A collective calling themselves a Group for a Different Medicine (GDM), which grew within SHC, stepped forward to organize some aspects of the Workers' Health Centre (WHC). In 2017 I spoke with two members of the GDM, Ilektra Bethymouti and Frosso Moureli, who shared some of their collective's writings with me. At its core, their aim has been to move beyond providing conventional medicine for free. Instead, they want to overcome elements that are broken in dominant approaches to healthcare. To paraphrase:

> Current medicine separates
> - the person from their environment
> - the doctor from the patient
> - the body from the psyche
> - the body into many parts
>
> ... without ever putting them together again.

Accordingly, the WHC is animated by the same spirit of the parent Social Solidarity Health Center, challenging the hierarchy in conventional doctor-patient relationships. The patient is renamed an incomer (the Greek word for patient has connotations of feebleness) and incomers are encouraged and empowered to become a member of the clinic's governing assembly, to participate actively in matters of their health and to connect it with the health of their community. In the writing of the GDM the incomer's active participation in their own health and community *is itself* a central form of their health treatment. The healing begins by undoing the subordination and alienation they have experienced not only in capitalist society but also in the conventional medical system where they are typically seen either as a body, or a worker, or a person, but never as all three at once. The GDM write: "we aspire to a medical science that does not simply perceive the symptom but treats it as part of the human being as a whole. Namely as a physical/psychic/social unity—like the two sides of a coin—that cannot be possibly separated."

Based on these principles, The WHC began to put into action new practices. The four "endeavors" I explain below were carefully narrated to me by Frosso Moureli, a psychiatrist and psychotherapist, who has been involved in the SHC, the WHC and the GDM from their inception. In all four endeavors, we can see (in an unprecedented way) what happens when neither the bank nor the state nor the doctor is not the boss of a healthcare facility. When healthcare is taken out of the exclusive clutches of jealous "experts," medicine can become cooperatively creative and can actually produce multiple forms of mutually reinforcing "health": physical, emotional, social, communal and relational.

The four endeavors below may seem subtle, but are deeply significant. It's also worth mentioning that all the solidarity clinics are participatory democracies, so the GDM or any other group can't simply redesign a health system from scratch: it's a matter of compromise and experimentation.

Four Endeavors for a Different Medicine

1. The first endeavor was a new reception protocol at the Solidarity Health Center, to greet incomers in empowering ways. The goal was to begin to erode the fearful sublimation of authority that a person goes through when they enter conventional clinics as a patient. As an outsider, I imagine that when receiving free care there is a sense that a patient must gratefully and uncritically accept what they are given. But by helping new people understand

how the clinic worked, inviting them to be active and ask questions, the reception team encouraged incomers to be discerning and proactive about their own needs and interests, and also to internalize the values of the clinic (solidarity and its power) and get involved.

2. The second endeavor was to hold what they called "joint sessions," a regular meetup for healthcare practitioners and incomers at the Solidarity Clinic meant to put providers and receivers of care together in a new context and so erode the invisible divide and hierarchy.

3. The third endeavor was organizing group meetings for people who were affected by diabetes. For ten months, anyone was welcome to come into the group to talk about the entire cycle of the disease. This group's purpose was to co-create a safe social space to make connections between the disease and their personal history, living conditions, social environment and personal health care management. The members of the group spoke about their own needs, medical or personal. Doing so built a community of trust, care, knowledge sharing and support. At the end of ten months all the members had their diabetes well in control, and two had made major life changes.

4. The final endeavor, still under development, is something the group called an "integrative model," and it is what drew me to Greece. Explained to me first by Ilektra and then by Frosso, this model is based on a different idea of health, authority, care and expertise.

In this model, the incomer meets with three health practitioners at the same time on their first 90-minute visit: a general physician, a psychotherapist and a social worker or (if no social worker is available) a non-practitioner volunteer. The social worker (or volunteer) leads the incomer through a survey, called a health card, of optional questions covering their mental, emotional and physical health, but also their broader situation, including their family life, living conditions, work, nutrition and sleep patterns; all are considered important aspects of health in a broad, holistic sense. As Frosso put it, they are trying to make *a hologram* of every person: a clear three-dimensional image of health. This image not only benefits the care-givers, who now know the whole person, but also the incomer who can see themselves and their challenges more interdimensionally.

The health card, which is attached to the incomer's medical file, also includes a family tree, which tracks the quality of relationships and matters of heredity. At follow-up meetings the practitioners and the incomer reflect on all the physical, social and psychological information on the health card. Here, the group helps the incomer take steps toward treatment, and helps them develop a plan to do so in a way where they can manage and get support for their own healing. Key questions include: What does the incomer need in order to thrive? What actions can they take, in terms of family, work and money, to help them to feel healthy? I imagine that a future question might be: what social movement might they join to experience the healing capacities of solidarity? When I last spoke to Frosso the group was working on what to do after this initial incomer meeting. As of January 2018, they had seen 50 incomers in this way.

"Our" Crisis, Our Bodies

I wanted to take something back to my context of the US. If their crisis is also our crisis, then their work can help us, and their learning can be our learning. As a person who had never thought critically about healthcare, the experiments I had encountered in Greece made me dream of a vast reimagining of what health care could be, especially in a country where so many of us are denied care or driven into bankruptcy by it. While I don't think that American doctors will volunteer en masse as they did in Greece, and while free clinics in squatted buildings are unlikely to survive the punitive arm of the state (regulation, legislation, insurance bureaucracy or police raids), there is so much we can learn from the kind of medicine that is being practiced at the Social Solidarity Clinic.

During my visit to Greece, I wondered how much of the work of the clinics could also be done without doctors or specialists, without training and without certification. How much of the success of the free clinic was about providing basic human care, compassionate attention and a safe space to ask questions? This, in contrast to the conventional "clinical," bureaucratic, service-oriented and hierarchical model we're used to and have been taught to value. As I sat in the Solidarity Clinic waiting rooms, talked with doctors, observed assemblies and accompanied incomers as they met with practitioners, I learned that most of the care given didn't need professional expertise—it was human connection, the provision of empathy and attention within what otherwise feels like an uncaring and alienating world where "the crisis" becomes lodged in the body.

Like Andromeda's copper rings that kill bacteria without washing, 99 percent of the time people can help each other; they don't need medical training to provide the preventative care and problem solving that most people need to persist. Like Andromeda the microbiologist's claims this figure is an overstatement. I'm not proposing that we don't need expertise at all. But so much of what produces "health," in a holistic sense, we can create without it, together.

Based on my study of the Workers' Health Center, I am striving to create a platform for collective healthcare, accountability and solidarity that can serve anyone falling between the widening cracks of highly regulated capitalist police states, regardless of where they live. I have been inspired to do so not only by my visit to Greece, but also by the conditions of my life and the lives of my friends: we have all been made itinerant and exiled from our physical communities of support by the forces of capitalism, including gentrification, the gig economy, racism and changing life circumstances. We've been denied access to quality, reliable healthcare, but have also come to rightly distrust conventional healthcare systems which are isolating, individualizing and often toxic. We need another model.

VĀG
ABO
NDS

Is this the End or is this the Beginning? A Four-Part Course in Social Holography

The following is a short course to prepare us to become holograms, which is to say to develop and practice *The Hologram* as a method of organized social care and collective liberation. It is the residue of a four-part *Hologram* workshop designed and delivered once per week by Cassie Thornton and Lita Wallis online with a group of 28 participants from around the world in April 2020 during the Covid-19 lockdown.

The objective of the course was to create a laboratory to experiment with building social and communicative skills and practices that would be useful to starting and maintaining a Hologram. The group practiced specific verbal and somatic communication skills and experimented with vulnerability, trust and cooperation, all contextualized in a theoretical framework. Throughout the four-week course, all 28 participants attempted to use the personal pronoun "we" when describing their own or another person's experiences, thoughts or feelings.

New Patterns for a Post-Capitalist Now

At its broadest and most ambitious scale *The Hologram* is intended as an open-source, peer-to-peer, viral social technology for dehabituating humans from capitalism. Capitalism is not only an economic system, it's a cultural and social system as well, which deeply influences how we relate to one another, how we interact, how we imagine ourselves and one another, even how we talk and feel. *The Hologram* relies on us disentangling ourselves from capitalism's influence, and that of white supremacy, colonialism, (cis hetero) patriarchy and other systems of domination, and it also helps us in this untangling.

For this reason, in addition to the social practices involved in forming groups of four and doing the work of "social holography," *The Hologram* is also a delivery mechanism for ideas about how we can reinvent our world by developing new daily habits that incorporate radical re-interpretations of these four themes: Trust, wishes, time, and patterns.

The following is an abbreviated set of materials from the April 2020 workshop to help readers reflect on and transform their habits and approaches to these important themes. This is meant to be group work, but many of us are alone right now, so we hope that these ideas and practices may inspire or contribute to how we already imagine and organize our care labor. Each unit includes a brief series of reflections, as well as several exercises we can do to prepare for practicing *The Hologram* model in the future.

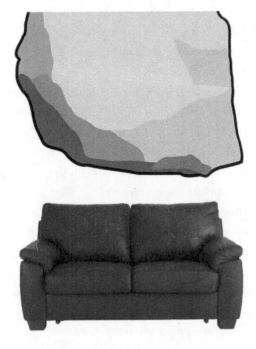

"Everything always works out."

In 2014 I went to a payday lender in my neighborhood to borrow $750 to pay rent and buy groceries. It took me two years and $1600 to pay that debt. I did not ask a friend for the money I needed because I could not accept that anyone I trusted would want to help me, or that they could afford to help me. I didn't know when or how I would be able to pay back the loan, and I wouldn't want anyone to have to share my precarity with me. I also didn't know whom I could explain my situation to without feeling ashamed. I didn't want to undergo a negotiation that could expose my private economic failure, or to invite someone else to expose their private financial status to me. Instead, I went to a storefront debtshop I knew was hideously exploitative and extortionate and asked a stranger for money from behind thick glass. These days, I could do it over an app without seeing another human being, assuming that I could afford my phone bill.

As more people fall below the poverty line or live in a state of constant economic emergency, "fringe" financial service companies have developed a multitude of easy and anonymous systems to offer fast loans through impersonal systems that sanitize exchange. This level of automation may alleviate a feeling of shame for needing financial help, but it also eliminates the potential for experiencing care or practicing negotiation. There are a million ways to get quick money *without feeling like a burden* on any one. In an age where we are taught we can't trust anyone but ourselves, and when asking another to trust us is deeply uncomfortable, the quality of social bonds, and even our ability to imagine and create those social bonds, corrodes. This doesn't just happen in the debt industry but across a world reshaped by capitalism as we're constantly told to trust corporations and politicians we know are ripping us off just so we don't have to learn to trust ourselves and one another. I have identified three of the toxic lessons teach us that we need to unlearn if we are going to build a post-capitalist future.

Bad support

Bad support, which is usually given by corporations but also sometimes by austerity-minded governments and institutions, begins when you're led to believe that you are receiving some kind of help that will allow you to thrive, but then this "help" reveals itself to take more than it ever gives. Often and obviously this comes in the form of extortionate debt, a life-line that's actually a noose. But it can come in other forms too: a dream job that turns into a nightmare, etc. The worst part of this lesson is that it trains us to expect bad support or unexpected punishment when we are most in need, so we may start to avoid seeking any kind of support and believe in self-reliance *which is impossible for a cooperative species.* Worse still, we may reproduce this pattern when we are asked for support, *because it is all we know*: we become bad support for others. This may happen because we fear our support for others will be bad and so we never learn to offer it. Or when we offer support, we're so scared of making a mistake that we overdo it and exhaust ourselves. Or offer non-transformative support that maintains the status quo.

The atrophy of the sharing muscle

If we can only accept help from corporations or institutions, we lose the skills and practices involved in asking for and offering help from people in our community. Having relationships where our central resources are carefully shared is fundamentally intuitive to humans, a cooperative species. But like language, which must be learned, these practices are far from innate. They take energy, time and practice. Central resources include housing, money and our skilled labor. Sharing them requires lifelong practices of communication and negotiation. Unfortunately, since sharing is so devalued in this society, we are led to believe that it's easy or automatic. But when we do not actively practice sharing our resources we lose the muscles needed to do so, and we may even forget that this kind of hardcore interdependence is possible or desirable. Indeed, it can seem like a threat. Attention and care are also central resources and, while we all have the capacity to produce and receive them, it's not automatic and requires practice and structure.

Failienation

If we don't have experiences sharing resources, or sharing our stories of struggle in an unfair financial and social landscape, we may feel like we alone are failures: failienation.

If we feel that our inability to thrive is our personal responsibility and that we alone have failed (instead of realizing that the systems of support have failed all of us), we may not want to share our story or ask for help because we assume that we would be a burden on other people (if we assume they are not feeling like failures themselves). This is a self-defeating defense mechanism and often manifests in everyday life as being anti-social or even incurious toward others.

It's vital to recognize that falienation also affects the fortunate. Let's say that you've worked out a way to survive well enough in this brutal financial landscape and your material needs are covered or exceeded. This can be alienating in part because your security comes largely from your ability to purchase what you need, rather than relying on others, and partly because you are living in a society where some people's comfort comes at the expense of others. In a system where only some are permitted to thrive we come to resent one another in all directions, which maximizes distrust and makes it even harder to learn to share central resources.

Learning to Trust Ourselves Again for the First Time

The Hologram is a social technology to rebuild the social trust that has been dissolved by living in and with Capitalism. Decades of neoliberalism and austerity have taught us that our health is our personal responsibility. Most governments' responses to the current pandemic have allowed whatever trust we had in them to look out for our welfare to melt like salt in hot water, and now we have to gargle with this stuff. Many people have lost their jobs and their ability to pay rent, and the state (in most cases) has done little to nothing to support them. The last crystals of trust in society have dissolved.

This is (always already!) the time to ask: How do we imagine our own care, before or during an emergency, within a set of completely unstable conditions?

The Hologram creates a space where it is possible to have repeated social experiences of commitment and attention from people who are doing so without economic motivation. It is a practice-ground where these invaluable experiences can be given and received, accepted and sanctioned. The assumption of *The Hologram* is that we can train ourselves to trust each other and to trust ourselves.

We are in for the fight of our lives in the years to come to save the world from capitalism, but whatever post-capitalism we hope to build can't be magicked into existence and will not be handed to us. To better be able to join the struggle for it, and to prepare to take our place within it as cooperative, interconnected animals, we need to practice new forms of trust. It is simple as an idea and much harder as a practice because we have all been taught toxic lessons. So, experimenting with sharing hardcore resources, starting with time and energy, may feel uncomfortable or dangerous. It is only with repetition and persistence that we can "remember" or rebuild some of these skills that we had to shed to survive a hyper individualistic financial landscape. We believe this is a practice that anyone can participate in.

Questions for Consideration

- Can we do this without experts?
- Can we do this without space?
- Can we do this without money?
- Can we do this without stability?
- Can we do this when we are all a little sick?

- Can we do this when we have been taught that we can only trust experts?
- Can we do this when we don't even trust ourselves?

Activity 1

1. On paper make a T chart. On the left side write a list of who you call when you are really stuck but need to make a decision.
2. On the right side list all the people who come to you for the same reason.
3. Which side has more people?
4. What's the difference between the people who you trust, and those who trust you?
5. What would it take to help the people who need support to be able to become people who you could go to for support? Or, what would help your supporters become better at what they do for you? And, what would make you better at offering support?
6. For each person, and in relationship to you, consider the following
   - Boundaries (positive and negative)
   - Courage (yours and theirs)
   - Skills (yours and theirs)
7. Based on your considerations, circle the three people you might approach to be your triangle, if you were to be a hologram.
8. Based on your considerations above, circle the three people whom you might learn from if they were a hologram and you were in their triangle.

2. WISHES

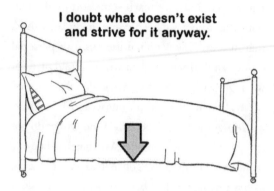

**I doubt what doesn't exist
and strive for it anyway.**

Nothing makes me feel more alive than helping other people solve their problems. It makes me feel powerful, useful, connected and of service. It is necessary work, and it uses all my skills: deep attention, creative problem solving, vengeful empathy. But the focus on problems, which tend to arise in moments of (or approaching) crisis, means we can never plan very far into the future. Because most of my loved ones have very little money or security, we use chewing gum to plug the leaks only long enough to get us to the next disaster. This is the way most of us must live right now at the intersection of many multi-layered crises. We feel we can't dare to wish for anything in case it distracts us from the crisis at hand, as if wishing were an unacceptable indulgence. Sybille Peters is an artist who has theorized wishes as a fundamental part of rigorous research practices. If it wasn't for her work, I think I would be unable to use the word without rolling my eyes at the same time.

But what if we challenge ourselves to see through these emergencies and to go toward our wishes despite all the holes in our boats? After all, those holes are only going to get plugged, not really fixed, until we reach some sort of destination. Right now, we keep going in circles. I think that in some way we often use our own personal crises as a distraction when we are afraid of what we might wish for. So long avoided in the name of survival, we may not know our wishes, or we may not recognize them, especially if our wishes do not comply with what is on offer. We may feel like our wishes are not utterable, or that we don't deserve to have wishes, either because we're obviously a failure or because we already have too much. We may feel that our wishes don't make sense in a capitalist context. We may have never seen a good wish come to fruition. We may feel that our wishes are too weird or individualistic or simple to talk about in the company of people we respect, who appear to have much better wishes. Or maybe there simply isn't time to talk about this bullshit, which will keep us from the work of survival ... and will inevitably lead us to more disappointment. Making wishes in the apocalypse feels risky. But maybe the apocalypse in one way came from too many neglected wishes.

If all our Crises are Connected, then all our Wishes are Conspiring

I have a sixth or seventh sense that your deepest wishes may not be that different from mine. It takes time to be able to understand and articulate them. Even if I knew my wishes I may not be able to describe them because there aren't many opportunities to practice that type of thinking or speaking. I don't think wishes can live in a vacuum. Wishes are social. We create them together as we survive and learn what we want to escape and what we want to go toward. We hold them together.

It is hard to wish for what we haven't yet seen. And what if all we know is that we don't want any more of what we have been exposed to? This is very scary. We may sometimes fixate on solving problems as a way to avoid having dangerous wishes. Our wishes might demand that we abolish this society and create a new one, one that can meet all our wishes. An honest wish can make it hard or even impossible to continue to participate in this society. How are you going to go to work for minimum wage if you know it is completely disconnected from what you want or believe in? What if the only way to meet your wish in our present society is to do something or benefit from something you hate? Me too. But the dangerous wishes are there, under the bed like a monster designed by you, for you.

The Wish Beneath the Wish

As a member of a triangle in a Hologram there is an opportunity to see someone's struggles in relationship to their spoken or unspoken wishes. In isolation it can be really hard to remember our larger goals and wishes, especially when we have learned to be placated with bad news, untrustworthy information and massively unequal and unfair living conditions. This project asks all participants to uphold a forceful optimism: we will survive

better together. We can create a world where our
wishes are contingent on each other's fulfillment,
not on endless competition. And we suspect that
the wishes we each have, when put together, can
give us the energy and sustenance we need to
engage in the ongoing crisis. We can solve each
other's problems as we go toward our dreams,
and getting closer to what we want will give us the
energy to continue to deal with the never-ending
list of emergencies.

The Hologram is one methodology for unpacking
our wishes; because I suspect that there is always a
wish hiding below our wishes.

For example, you wish for a house on a nice
piece of land, somewhere quiet and beautiful.
Many people do. But the first level of unpacking
includes the following questions: Why might you
wish for that? Had you been taught to want that?
What are you reproducing? Who else benefits from
that wish? Who suffers at the hand of this wish?

Is another layer beneath that? *It's important not
to get caught up in beating ourselves up for our wishes, but
to ask deeper questions, to understand what they are trying
to say.* What kind of person is constructed by this
wish? A taxpayer? A head of household? A gar-
dener? A home decorator? A mother? Does the
wish produce the character that you need and want
to become, in the conditions that we are living in?

What is below this wish? Is it that you seek
stability? Do you desire safety? Do you want to
experience natural beauty every day? Do you
want to ensure your access to food? Do you want
to be able to create a safe space for others in your
community?

There is always a multitude of wishes below the original wish. Maybe it's wishes all the way down. By looking below the wish without shame, we may be able to understand what it is that is non-negotiable, and how we can meet the wish without compromising our values. Because if we fail to question and complicate our wishes, most of us at some point will have a hard time striving to meet our unquestioned wish within a system that is actually killing us or others so that only a handful can have their wish fulfilled, if indeed it is their wish and not a proxy.

The work of excavating our wishes, of carefully and optimistically discovering our wishes beneath our wishes, and the ways our wishes are connected, is some of the work we can do in *The Hologram*.

Questions for Consideration

- What have you been taught to want?
- What do you wish you wanted?
- What do you want not to want?
- What do you pretend to want?
- What if you do not want what is on offer?
- What do you want?

Activity 2

Move your arms as if you are swimming freestyle, extending one, then the other, in constant motion in big circles, elbows pulling the arms above your shoulders.

As you swim, imagine yourself in a vast ocean. Night is falling and a storm is coming. You can't see the shore, so you use your intuition to orient you. Project yourself in that direction, and swim vigorously so that the motion will naturally put your breath into rhythm. Continue for seven minutes.

Now, make a list of the three biggest challenges you currently face. If you overcame each of these challenges, recovered your energy and realized you could safely make a wish, what would that wish be?

What would it feel like to have support confronting these challenges? How would the three people you listed in Activity 1 offer you the kind of support you need to get to the wish? Create an invitation to your triangle that describes the type of support you would like to receive if they would join your Hologram.

3. TIME

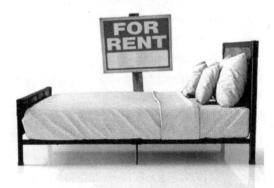

I don't have enough time to imagine something better.

We Don't Have Time for This!

Time is the number one barrier to participation in *The Hologram* with good reason: we guard our time against anything that could chip away at the hours and energy we are made to dedicate to work, pleasure or survival. Under capitalism, time has become the most valuable commodity we have, outside of our body. As capitalism becomes more and more punishing and demanding, we have less and less time to imagine a different future. We've even heard people say that the ability to "imagine" something outside of work and survival is a "privilege."

But, as we've already seen, capitalism is, among other things, a brilliant technology of weaponized avoidance. For our purposes, it helps us avoid at least three basic truths:

1. Humans are fundamentally cooperative and interdependent.
2. We live on land and are part of that land.
3. We will die.

What would it mean to live without forgetting these truths? Our time would be very different. If we focused on learning how to cooperate without coercion we would have to reorganize what we produce, how we produce it, and why. If we acknowledged that we lived on land, and that land was alive, and that we are a part of it, we would laugh at the absurdity of the concept of private property. If we lived our whole lives embracing the knowledge that we will die we would better consider future generations as we made decisions. We might spend our whole lives carefully considering our uses of materials and time, knowing that our collective material and social traces produce the next generations' world. We would recognize that the now-dead once did so for our benefit. We would know that, when we die, we become each other's soil.

If we remembered and believed these three truths how would we spend our time? What would our relationships look like? Where would we live and how? What would be our "work" and how would we be valued?

How and Why *The Hologram* Wastes Your Time

The Hologram aims to train us to create and live in a post-capitalist future, when work (as in labor exploited for a wage) is abolished. We will still need to cooperate, but in new ways, motivated by the above truths, not the need for someone else to profit and for us all to compete. When liberated from being confined to a "job," how would we express and share our passions, skills, powers and dreams? In post-capitalism, we will all contribute our time and energy, but likely in very different ways.

Today, for many of the readers of this text, participation in *The Hologram* feels like an impossible time commitment in an already over-busy life, but this is exactly why you should try it. It is a practice for liberating time, though it also takes time. It does so for participants at all stages. The following walks you through three phases of one's participation.

You are the Hologram

We suggest that you who are reading this begin participating in *The Hologram* by inviting three people to act as your triangle. You, the hologram, facilitated a conversation where your group decides who should play what role (who is in charge of asking about and holding social, mental/emotional and physical health information). Next, you decide together how long this experiment will last. When will you meet, and for how long?

> *Sample plan: You may meet on the first Wednesday of every third month, or on the day after the seasons change, four times per year. You may start with a one-year commitment to this process, or something else. Perhaps you meet for two hours each session. This seems possible, right?*

Consider what this would do to your sense of time. *The Hologram* is an impractical and life-giving social planning technology. How far into the future are you able to imagine right now? What in your life will be in place in three months, in six months, in two years? It may be scary to look into the future. If it isn't, you may be delusional. In such an unpredictable time, it is hard to know what will remain of our current lives in the future. But if we don't begin to construct some ideas and practices that will shape our future in ways that serve us then tech corporations, banks, right-wing governments and other anti-social saboteurs will have a complete run of it.

The Hologram asks us to put a formal agreement together with people in our community that will extend, outlandishly, into the future. Beyond the multiple overlapping crises that we will face, we can make commitments that structure our future selves and give us a sense of belonging, no matter where we are. Making a decade-long plan with your friends seems like heresy while we work daily to survive a deranged and predatory economy, alone and alienated, unable to prepare for the next crisis. This is exactly why you may want to commit to spending a few years with *The Hologram*, with your triangle.

You care for your caretakers

Being cared for, and being a hologram, is never a one-way street. In order to receive care from other people it is crucial that you help ensure that those people are cared for. It is not optional, it is required. So, in one of your early meetings you, the hologram, must help your triangle consider the timeline in which they will become holograms and develop their own triangles of support.

> *Sample plan: During your second Hologram meeting, the hologram proposes that each of the members of her triangle begin to invite three people to be their triangle/supports, to make themselves a hologram. It is agreed upon that this will take place before the next meeting. You talk together about what would make for a good triangle member.*

As a practicing hologram, you have created and fulfilled a role for yourself that does not yet exist in our society. In this post-capitalist "job," in being vulnerable and open to receiving care, you are the expert and the teacher. No one knows more than you about what makes you healthy. Just like starting a new job, you have to create a workspace that is appropriate for the work you need to do. So, it is your job to arrange and coordinate the triangle. Under capitalism, this kind of work is not valued. We value it in *The Hologram*.

If time is money, then being the hologram, or participating in a Hologram, is like burning money. It's a sacrifice that reveals your divestment from the accelerationist value system. Through the sacrifice we become different animals that can survive and see beyond the current economic landscape. If we use this collective work as an excuse to disentangle from capitalism's way of valuing our time, and of valuing us, we may begin to see what we are or what we could become without it. How would you identify yourself if you never had to have a "job" again? What would you do all day if you didn't need to "work" in order to live? How would you value your time if it was disconnected from money? How would you cooperate and contribute if you could do so in a way and in conditions you chose? What would your role be in the post-work, post-capital future? What would a satisfying day feel like?

You become triangular

When the three members of your triangle each have transitioned to holograms with their own triangle supporting them, it is your chance to transform into a caretaker within someone else's project.

Sample plan: in your third meeting, you, as hologram, inquire if the three members of your triangle have established themselves as holograms. If so, you can ask for their help to become a member of a triangle for a new Hologram. Maybe the new hologram is a co-worker or friend you've told about the project, somebody who understands the point of the project is solidarity, not charity. As a future member, you shouldn't organize a new hologram's triangle for them, but you can help and offer suggestions. It is important that each hologram take the initiative and responsibility to organize their Hologram and triangle.

Questions for Consideration

- In the world we want to create, how will we value our time? Do we measure it? Do we even know it is there? What would we do all the time? How will we value ourselves and each other?
- What will your post-capitalist "job" be?

Activity 4

Write, walk, think or draw as you imagine ten years in the future. If that is overwhelming, here are some questions to help you distill your thoughts.

- What do you know about yourself and your situation at that time?
- What do you not know about yourself and your situation at that time?

- What do you look forward to taking place between now and then?
- What do you fear may take place between now and then?
- What can you plan?
- What will make you feel prepared to handle what is coming?
- What do you wish for yourself?
- Why? What's underneath that desire?
- What do you wish for you and for everyone?
- How can you be best prepared to make that possible?

* Please do not avoid the global, political and environmental situation, and your connection to community and society.

Activity 5

How did you stay together with your triangle for ten years? Write, walk, think or draw as you imagine ten years in the future as a hologram. If that is overwhelming, here are some questions to help you distill your thoughts.

Imagine that you found three people to be in your Hologram, and that you stayed together for ten years. They each had their own Hologram. You were also part of someone else's triangle, maybe two people's. There is a sense of trust between people, but also something more specific. These are new kinds of relationships that are formal, sustainable and warm. You feel like you are part of something that is different than your previous experiences of family, friendships, work relations, social movements or professional caretakers. When you are caring for your hologram, you feel like you are part of something larger.

- How did you stay together with your triangle for ten years?
- What skills did you personally develop to make this possible?
- What are the benefits, to you, of having been in this group for so long?
- What are the challenges you already faced together with your triangle?
- What kinds of processes did you have to develop, and skills did the group have to learn, in order to do this?
- How does it feel to imagine having this role in the Hologram, versus not having it?

4. PATTERNS

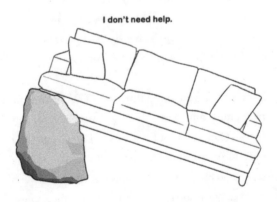

I don't need help.

Is This the End or is This the Beginning?

Whether actually or ideologically, the things we relied on to help us survive turned out not to work in the ways many of us hoped they would: the financial system, medical system, government. Long before Covid-19 a lot was crumbling (and the effects of the crumbling was always worse for people outside of white heteronormativity), and now none of us can avoid it.

According to an abolitionist framework, whenever broken systems crumble we have two types of work to do. One is to support the destruction of what isn't working and perhaps mourn its loss. The other is to create cooperative systems and ways of living that will work in the future and allow us to thrive. Now and in the coming months many people will experience a kind of end of the world: we will lose loved ones, jobs, houses, aspirations and a sense of "normal" as well as many things we thought were necessary. But maybe we will also realize that so much of what we felt was normal and necessary wasn't working for us, individually or collectively, but we had been made too busy trying to survive to notice. For some of us the Covid-19 lockdown was the moment when the band-aid was ripped off and we had an excuse to start fresh. We can demolish in the night and rebuild in the morning.

We are able to reproduce our lives within capitalism and other systems by forming habits of behavior, of thought, of hope, of fear and of relationship. These habits also do their part to reproduce those broader systems. These systems keep us so busy and on edge of survival (physical, emotional, social) that we rarely have the consistency of time to examine let alone change our habits, even if they don't actually serve us well.

From within the lockdown and after we have a chance to change some of our habits and patterns, so we don't have to go back to an expensive and violent normal. It's interesting to think about the world we want to live in in a theoretical way, but now we have a chance to experiment with how we live our daily lives and how we value ourselves and each other, and let those practices define the future.

Of course, contrary to the new age, self-help industry's suggestion, simply believing something doesn't change reality, and that kind of individualism will only reproduce capitalism. Organizing and organization will be required, and we have the fight of our lives ahead of us. But a revolution like the one we need will not come about or stick unless we, as its participants, transform ourselves together. Changing our patterns and habits alone won't liberate us, but it will help us prepare for liberation, and for the world we will have to build.

Prediction, Cognition and Emotion

Predictions are basically the way your brain works. It's business as usual for your brain. Predictions are the basis of every experience that you have. They are the basis of every action that you take. In fact, predictions are what allow you to understand the words that I'm speaking as they come out of my … .

Lisa Feldman Barrett

Neuroscientist Lisa Feldman Barrett explains that, while we typically assume prediction is a complex and advanced mental function, it's actually at the core of how neurotypical humans think, and is deeply connected with our emotions. As we experience the world, and even in our dreams, our brains are constantly making predictions about what will happen next, based on our past experiences. "Predictions are primal," she theorizes. "They help us to make sense of the world in a quick and efficient way. So your brain does not react to the world. Using past experience, your brain predicts and constructs your experience of the world." This all happens at lightning speed, outside of our conscious mind. A lot of our emotional life stems from this: when our past experience has shaped our brain to expect something good from an experience we can be pleased, calm and satisfied when our predictions about that experience are verified. The opposite is also true: We can become distraught, angry or hostile when our predictions are contradicted.

Ultimately, then, the way our brain experiences and makes sense of the world is through a combination of habits, patterns and emotions. This agrees with a lot of many people's common experiences of feeling trapped in cycles or stuck in a rut, although we also need to consider that not all brains work in the same way. When we provide support to friends or family, it's not just about commiseration but helping them recognize patterns and unhelpful emotional responses. If that's all true, and if the brain is as elastic and changeable as we know it is, then we can repattern and transform the brain, and ourselves, by creating and sustaining new habits and patterns.

What happens when everyone, at the same time, experiences the need to create new habits, when the pressures within which we created our old patterns disappear?

De-habituation From Capitalism

So many of our patterns and habits have been formed as ways to survive within the pressures of capitalism, but in this moment many of those pressures have evaporated. There is a rare opportunity to experiment and build new habits and patterns.

For example, within capitalism we have habituated ourselves to imagine that when we receive something, even if it's a life-giving object or service, we are obligated to reciprocate something considered to be of equal value, whether it is for chewing gum or toothpaste, massage or rent. Maybe the impulse for fairness comes from a good place, but in many ways this habit is deeply unhelpful. For instance, most of our most important relationships, with friends or parents, are necessarily unequal in terms of the time, energy and "resources" one of us commits relative to the other. We have programmed ourselves to imagine that you must give something equivalent to what you receive, but that's not always appropriate. Sometimes people give and they don't want anything in return. In fact, this inclination is absolutely essential to society and life. It works because, as the saying goes, what goes around comes around: giving without the need for reciprocal exchange is something we all benefit from and we all do, but not always with the same people. But in spite of the fact this is central to our lives, it's hard to see and trust because our brains are so patterned by our experience of capitalism that insists that all value comes from competitive or at least equivalent exchange. We feel compelled to give, or even guilty if we don't reciprocate. This is a big, gross pattern.

My friend in Palestine told me that until recently her mom had never bought food. She had only grown it or raised it or was given it. To spend money on food was, for her, absurd. I have only ever bought food. This made me consider how deeply limiting my experience and patterns have been, formed as they are in a transactional culture.

Creating New Patterns

The Hologram necessarily relies on and makes possible the creation of new patterns. When three people turn their care and attention on one it fundamentally challenges many of the habits we have formed to survive under capitalism. We cannot change our habits alone. It is partly for this reason that we consider the hologram a teacher and not just a subject of care: when she allows herself the vulnerability and generosity to accept help in identifying, breaking and forming new patterns, she offers an opportunity for the whole triangle to learn how such a process might work. Even accepting such care, or learning to provide it, necessarily means we have to break many patterns and habits. In *The Hologram* we quite literally rewire our brains, together.

Here are some examples of patterns we transform in *The Hologram*.

Complicating reciprocity

You receive care but you don't give back directly
to the person or people who gave it to you. There
is no equal exchange, tit for tat. There's a chance
here to reprogram our ideas about reciprocation
and transaction within a caring network of people,
when we know that care is being well distributed
and that reciprocation is always happening, and
when it's no longer a mystery how to do it well.
Importantly, *The Hologram* as a distributed social
technology, "works" when many hologram groups
are interlinked, so that reciprocity isn't a two-way
street but a network: those who provide care do, in
the end, also receive it, but from others.

Learning to see each other's patterns

This is the primal idea of *The Hologram*: even
after a short time, but especially after a long time
(ten years), a triangle is likely to be able to see
a hologram's patterns and help her move past
them if they do not serve her. There is something profoundly powerful and transformative
about observing and identifying others' patterns
and they help us recognize our own patterns and
habits which, while they might be very different,
perhaps emerged from similar pressures and circumstances. This is one important reason why the
hologram is a teacher, not a patient.

Creating new patterns

Within *The Hologram* we have chances to think
about creating new patterns for each other. A lot
of us have had really shitty experiences receiv-

ing attention, care or commitment or asking for support. We build up psychic defense mechanisms based on these bad experiences, which makes it harder and harder to receive support. In *The Hologram* we have the opportunity to give ourselves and each other positive experiences of these things, outside of our family, friendship and professional commitments.

Activity 6

1. To give yourself healing hands, so you can heal anyone or anything, even time itself:
   - Rub the palms of your hands together briskly for three to five minutes.
   - Stretch your arms out to the sides, parallel to the floor, palms up, thumbs pointing back as if you are balancing a dish on each hand. Set a timer and do the "Breath of Fire" for three minutes: forcefully exhale from your nostrils in a rapid, rhythmic way (your body will automatically inhale between breaths). You can start by letting your tongue hang out and pant like a dog, then close your mouth and keep breathing through your nose.
   - After three minutes, inhale and hold the breath in and, with your arms still out to your sides, bend your wrists so your palms are facing out (away from the body), as if you were pushing out the walls on either side of you. Feel the energy in the center of the palms flowing to your entire body. Exhale and relax the breath.

- Rub your hands together again for two minutes and continue Breath of Fire.
- Inhale and hold your breath. With your arms still out to the sides, bend your elbows so your hands are in front of your chest, like you're holding an eight-inch ball a few inches in front of your diaphragm, with the right hand flat on top of the ball and the left supporting it from below. Meditate on the exchange of energy between the palms of the hands for a few minutes.

2. Write a letter to one person who you would like to invite to be a member of your Hologram. You can use and revise the letter below, which was written by a participant in the project.

Sample Letter (written by Shawn Chua on May 4, 2020):

Dear ___,

I think I've shared with each of you about how I've been attending this workshop-experiment called *The Hologram*, and I'd like to invite you to be part of the Hologram that I'm hoping to establish. This sounds like an invitation to a cult, or a pyramid scheme, which structurally it does sort of resemble, but in a good way.

If you say yes you will be contributing to an experiment in peer to peer healthcare— with its roots in an integrative care model developed within the Social Solidarity Clinic movement in Greece, in response to the financial and migrant crisis. All our crises are connected, as we know more every day. You can read about the project here [*insert link*].

We've been having these conversations for a while now about scaffolding infrastructures of support, and how to take care of each other. I thought about how *The Hologram* might be an interesting model to operationalize that practice of care, and more importantly distributing that care work through this triangulation so that those who are offering that support may also find ways of mutually supporting one another. Again, this is in some ways not so different from what we're already doing for each other in an informal capacity, but I'm curious to see how this might be articulated differently through this model, and whether that can then be tessellated through the rest of our group.

If you agree you would join me in an online call for 90 minutes with Cassie, who will facilitate and observe.

- There will be a 15-minute introduction and discussion where we agree on guidelines for the session.
- The three of you will ask me questions to help me clarify my situation, and help me figure out how I really feel, emotionally, physically and socially about my current situation.
- There will be a 15-minute debrief.
- Afterwards Cassie will send you a survey to complete.

It would be amazing if you wanted to be involved, and I'd be happy to share more about the project if you need any clarifications. We can then arrange for a time and set it up with Cassie and see where this takes us.

REFLECTIONS

"When I Becomes We" by Elly Clarke
Artist and researcher

What happens when "I" becomes "we"?" "I" does already become "we" in quite a few aspects of life. In love, after a while. Families are also "we". And at work we talk about the firm that employs us as "we." Identities are described by "we." We are women. We are queer. We like drinking tea. We support key workers. We don't like Boris. Each "we" defines and combines us in various formations. But with "we," the boundary between "we" and "not-we" is placed at a further distance than when it's just I and you.

What happens, then, if "we" becomes, and is used as, a pronoun, even when someone is talking about their own individual experience? The Queen uses "we", but that's different, and about asserting a different kind of distance altogether. But what if we (non-royals) take "we" as a pronoun and use it as a radical act of collectivity, as a means and method of talking about difficult feelings, without pinpointing them onto one specific body? And what if, in the context of talking about these difficult feelings, we phase out the use of "I" altogether? What happens when

"I'm feeling anxious" becomes "we are feeling anxious?" Or "I had some issues come up about my past" to "we had some issues come up about our past?" How do we respond to "we" as a pronoun? How could it be used as part of a collective process of taking care and having care taken of us?

This was the premise of the four-week course for *The Hologram*, which was supposed to take place via the old-fashioned arrangement of bodies gathering in a room (at Furtherfield Gallery) but was forced online (to Zoom) due to the Covid-19 pandemic. An artist-led program exploring alternative, community-sourced methods of healthcare, the timing of the lockdown (the week before the first session) felt almost spookily serendipitous. With the ground shifting under our feet as we were confined to our homes, this group provided, for me at least, an anchor through which surprisingly embodied, in-depth conversations about things that really matter could take place, with people outside my regular circles.

"Holographic Hair" by Richard Houguez
Radical hairdresser

During *The Hologram* course I began to think about my approach to hairdressing as a different form of hologram. When someone sits in the hairdresser's chair there are three images present:

- What the person's hair used to look like (past self-image).

- What the person's hair looks like now (present self-image).
- How the person imagines their hair to appear after the haircut (future self-image).

Like the letter Q, hair is the line which grows out of the interior-personal space of our *self* and is touched by the exterior-social space of *culture*. Also like the letter Q, for queer people, telling their narratives and having them heard is both a powerful act and a question of safety.

A good haircut is when all of these images are integrated and tended to.

- A haircut to mark of change/event.
- A haircut to secure an income.
- A haircut to become adult.
- A haircut to change gender presentation.
- A haircut to experience grief.
- A haircut because of hair loss.
- A haircut to feel safe.
- A haircut to pass.
- A haircut as selfcare.
- A haircut to please someone else.
- A haircut as routine.
- A haircut as a treat.
- A haircut as a threat.
- A haircut as an exception.

The reasons people choose to cut their hair vary across the three images. It might be as a way of processing the past; it might be as a way of making space for the future. For some people it's a matter of healing (past), safety (present, future) or being inventive (future).

I was attracted to *The Hologram* course because of my experiences of the hairdresser-client relationship. It is widely recognized as an extraordinary relationship in that it can often span a long duration of time, be founded on trust, proximity and intimacy, yet be outside of models of family, friendship and romantic partnerships. It's an uneconomical relationship, in that it goes beyond expectations of transactions, just like friendships, yet strangely sits as a profession. This tension can be embarrassing, it can be pleasant.

Right now my empathy is tied up stylishly, tomorrow I might wear it down, free.

"Reflections from an Old Friend" by Tara Spalty

Therapist and Acupuncturist at Slow Poke Acupuncture in San Francisco and long-time collaborator on The Hologram

I am not used to being the focus of care. As a social worker in a community mental health clinic, my practice is "client focused." As an acupuncturist, and a harm reductionist, I am "patient-centered." It's not a strange story: I went to grad school for nearly eight years. I got a bunch of degrees, all in care-giving clinical professions, in an attempt to wrangle my natural interests and instincts into some financial viability in the hope of ending my precariousness, which didn't really work. Now, with Covid-19 we are all precarious.

There is no better time to put into practice this system that I was part of dreaming up. We need it. We need *The Hologram* to proliferate into a huge interconnected web and sustain. *The Hologram* course was an opportunity for me to practice *The Hologram* as the care receiver. This time I wanted to be a participant and not a presenter. I wanted to experience care only and refrain from giving. I knew it would be hard. I knew I would be distracted. I knew I would not do my homework. The series took place in the evening London time and so in San Francisco they always fell mid-morning, in the middle of my 9–5 work day. I felt like I had no time. As I am writing this, I have clinical assessments due that I need to complete for my social work job so that people can continue to receive services funded by the state. The sessions were interrupted by work and I missed the last one completely because of a migraine headache. I was exhausted and overwhelmed. Intimacy came quickly and then retreated. My paranoia and fear dissolved with even these small connections. I discovered that time is ours.

"We" by Lita Wallis
Co-facilitator

Grasped blindly for trust
In our isolations
Felt apprehension; a chesty fear pang
Asked the first question
Were interrupted
Bent our brains becoming a
We
Felt recognition

Examined our networks
Felt surrounded
like talking through water
exhausted
by the Therapeutic Industrial Complex
Were validated
We
Laughed
though it seemed impossible
Made sculptures of our emotions
when words wouldn't do
Threw ourselves about to 90s music
Breathed into hidden parts of ourselves
Wished

Struggled to find the right questions
Felt our fragility
Worried if our Hologram would be OK
left alone with our vulnerability
Wondered if we had done it right
Realized how much communication is felt
rather than heard
Listened

Realized that to survive
we have to bring our bodies with us
that the body cuts through
the bullshit learned by the mind
Became deeply connected
to tiny little squares full of humanity

Concocted some magic
to take back time from the bosses
Showed each other portraits:

each of us in lockdown
Predicted the future
Wondered how to close what We
had opened

Met with our barriers
Identified our shame
Were endlessly discerning
Wrestled with reciprocity
Saw ourselves
refracted in others
Felt united in our grief

Came back anonymous
Graduated as someone else
Entirely

The Practice

You are now ready to practice *The Hologram*. The following will offer you the basics. *The Hologram* remains a work in progress and is designed to be highly adaptable, so you are encouraged to change it and make it your own.

A *triangle* consists of three people who accept an invitation from a *hologram* to make a formal commitment to supporting her health by participating in seasonal meetings. In these meetings, each member of the triangle focuses on one of the three aspects of the hologram's health: physical, psychic, social. The task of each member of the triangle is to ask really good questions, help identify the hologram's patterns, and to support her with co-research and in-depth knowledge of her health when she needs to make big decisions.

The hologram's job is to facilitate a conversation with three people who have accepted her invitation to join the triangle. Unlike a patient being treated by a doctor, a hologram's role is like that of a teacher, helping the triangle to understand how she achieves her healthiest possible state and also recognize their own patterns, needs and wishes in contrast and conversation. The hologram shares her personal stories, her powers of communication and her well-articulated vul-

social care**

hologram*

physical care**

mental/emotional care**

*the hologram is a teacher

**triangle members are living medical records, not experts or advisors

nerability to teach the triangle how to care for and with her. She shows great respect and gratitude for the members of the triangle, and is also observant of their needs and desires, helping them to become better at offering useful questions.

This guide is written for holograms seeking to assemble triangles, but can also be used for triangle members seeking to find holograms.

How Will You Identify People
for Your Triangle?

No one knows what will work until it does. Invite people who make you feel comfortable, whose attention and care you enjoy and people who would like to do it for you.

Additionally, you might ask yourself these questions before deciding whom to invite:

- *Do I want the members to know each other?*
- *Do you want to include people you interact with regularly, or rarely?*
- *Do I want the members to all be local?*
- *Do I want to use this as an opportunity to develop new relationships, or to add a new layer to already existing relationships?*

Finally:

- *Oh no, I invited the wrong person out of cruel optimism about them or us and it was a bad idea. How do I get rid of them and pick a new person?!*

We recommend that you provide a trial period where you can experience the group for 1-2 sessions with the awareness among the group members that if the dynamic of the group is not great, there will be a chance to change its composition.

How Much Personal Information
do I Reveal?

You can decide. Whether we are online, on the phone, or at work, we are constantly warned to protect our privacy, but it is hard to keep in mind what we are guarding it from. The truth is that there are many types of predators who are seeking to profit from our information and our vulnerabilities, but those individuals and corporations are not here in this triangle. The goal is to learn to trust, and to want to share as much information as is necessary (but maybe not more) to help your triangle understand where you are coming from and where you may be going, so they can go there with you!

How do I Reciprocate?

Reciprocation is somewhat automatic in this project, but is not a one-for-one exchange, like paying for a hot-dog. For *The Hologram* project to really work every person must be a hologram as well as a member of someone else's triangle (not for someone in your triangle, though). The most important healing that you will receive from this project is when you successfully care for someone else. This networked reciprocation means that you will not be directly giving back what you receive from your triangle, but you will be a part of a larger cycle of reciprocation and the production of health, which can never be transactional. For this reason, it is the calling of each hologram to proactively help each member of her triangle find their own triangles and become holograms themselves. She must also seek to become part of a triangle for someone not in her triangle. The hologram can reciprocate by virally reproducing *The Hologram*.

**Every person must be
a hologram as well as
a member of someone
else's triangle.**

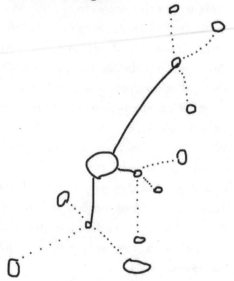

**Needing support
does not
make you weak.**

1. While it is possible that someone might have a medical or social work background, no one in a triangle is held to be an expert, and no one should pretend to be one. Being in a triangle is not about offering professional medical advice, it is about learning to ask supportive and transformative questions.

2. While *The Hologram* is about asking questions, the triangle members should not disappear their own stories, their needs or their wisdom. Triangle members are welcome to share anecdotes and stories from their lives that might help the hologram see her situation and clearly state her personal needs.

3. The triangle, with the hologram, will make group decisions and will structure the way the group meets.

4. When called upon in an emergency or a pressing situation the triangle can choose to show up to support the hologram as individuals or as a trio. The triangle becomes most active when the hologram needs to make a big decision. This is when all the triangles's accrued knowledge and notes, about the hologram become valuable. In an emergency, the triangle may support the hologram by providing in-person support, accompaniment to or coaching for important appointments and cooperative research. The goal of the triangle is to back the hologram to make good decisions.

What Role does Each Person Play?

A Hologram begins when the hologram and triangle agree to meet for a certain period of time at a certain frequency: once a week for a month; once a month for three months; around the solstices and equinoxes for two years; on the hologram's birthday for the rest of her life. It might make sense to begin with a shorter period of more frequent meetings then change later, or, if the group does not gel, to reform the triangle with new members. But a Hologram works best when practiced consistently over a long period of time to facilitate pattern recognition and transformation.

Within the given period, the three members of the triangle will select one area of focus in their meetings with the hologram. Each person will focus on asking questions and taking notes on one of the three zones of health: the physical (body), the psychic (mental, emotional, intellectual) and the social (relationships, work, money, housing).

Of course, these health zones are completely entangled and overlapping, and the conversation will be too. The important thing is that there is a member of the triangle to hold the awareness of each of the various zones of health, who can watch for patterns and feel when something is going well or not. We have not yet experimented with rotating roles within the triangle, but that is an option.

What if I Want to Quit? What if I Want
Someone Else to Quit?

58

The group should decide what to do in the event
that one of the members of the triangle wants
to quit. Because the project is about construct-
ing new experiences of trust and cooperation, it
is ideal if the group can adapt to support each
member to stay on in a healthy way. When that
cannot happen there needs to be an exit plan in
place, wherein the triangle member that exits is
replaced and that the new member is welcomed
into the group with care and patience. This exit
strategy should be discussed at the first meeting
of a Hologram.

How do we Keep Notes and Records?

This is up to your group (including the hologram)
to decide. The notes are a tool for the future,
to help you remember when something occurred
in the past and help everyone recognize patterns
and habits that can only become clear in hind-
sight. Well-labeled and organized notes can be
really useful. The notes can be shared among
everyone in the group, or just kept to individuals who wrote them. Since some people find
drawings and diagrams more useful we have built
some tools for how to organize and document
some patterns visually. Notes can go into a shared
folder online if you feel safe doing so, and we
are working on a safe space and system for that
to happen.

When do I Become a Hologram?

As we described in the Time section of the course, each member of the triangle will become a hologram. This means you will invite three people to make a triangle for you, and begin the process anew. We recommend that this happen shortly after your second or third successful meeting of the original Hologram. This is something you can and should discuss with the hologram you care for. Since you support her, it is in her best interest to support you in getting the care you need.

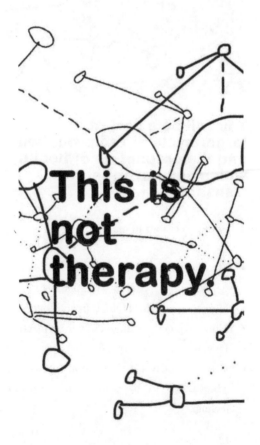

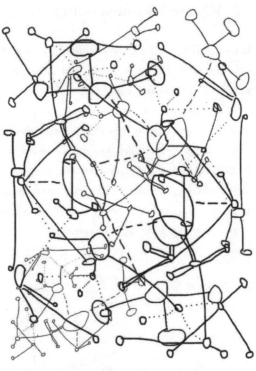

**You will be a part of a
larger cycle of reciprocation
and the production of health,
which can never be
transactional.**

Initial group decisions to make:

- How will the Hologram meet? (online? in person? where? and by what platform?)
- How long will this Hologram continue?
- How frequently will the Hologram meet?
- How long will each meeting be?
- How do you want the session to feel and what needs to happen to produce that feeling?

- How should a meeting begin? How should it end?
- How should notes be kept?
- What if someone wants to leave the group, or people can't work together?
- How will you deal with conflict?
- Can the triangle meet without the hologram?

VĀG
ABO
NDS

Wikipedia Entry
from the Future

From Wikipedia, the free post-internet
encyclopedia
(Redirected from Collective Health)

*This article is about the <u>Parafictional Social Practice Art
Project</u>. For other uses, see <u>Hologram (disambiguation)</u>*

The Hologram is a post-economic social organizing
system composed of post-secular social practices
that distribute attention, value and health to all
living beings. Initiated in the lead up to the <u>First
Global Pandemic</u> of 2020, *The Hologram* appeared
at first to be a viral art project, but soon revealed
itself to be a new <u>social technology</u> that assem-
bled voluntary participants into teams of four to
experiment with new models of health and social
care. It is widely acknowledged [citation needed]
that this social practice and storytelling strategy
came to comprise the original building blocks for
what has come to be known as the <u>post-money
economy</u> (PME): an attempt to organize and value
social and environmental resources based on their
ability to produce common health and life, rather
than private material wealth.

Due to its viral nature, which empowers practitioners to adapt to local and collective circumstances,
The Hologram and its <u>derivatives</u> have taken many
thousands of forms, but almost all are marked by
some or all of a suite of common features, notably:
the <u>stigmatization</u> of private property, the use of
the <u>Health Accumulation Index</u>, the autonomous
coordination of socially necessary labor, practices
of the <u>non-transactional exchange</u> of attention
and care, and <u>deschooling</u> from competition.

Since 2020, the practice has grown into what most
experts consider to be a fundamental element of
social life [citation needed], and it is popularly
believed, especially among its practitioners, to
be a tendency that has always been dormant in
the human experience. Most practitioners agree
that *The Hologram* was originally developed by
estranged artists (a now-obsolete "<u>job</u>" category)
mostly living in jurisdictions at the heart of the
former capitalist and colonialist <u>empires</u> (these
capital <u>"cities"</u> that had the highest rate of suicide,
addiction and depression before <u>The Great Iso-
lation</u>). Most origin stories hold that these artists
were organized by a figure named <u>Cassandra</u>,
though historians have questioned her influence
and even her existence. Today, the practice has
become a central element of the <u>Global Solidarity
Social Architecture</u> (GSSA).

Holograms do not simply produce the illusion of
depth but are truly three-dimensional.

Starting in 2020 *The Hologram* emerged as a practice and is today embedded in the daily life of at least 25 million people. However, when one includes its many derivative forms and unofficial uses, and the natural spread of its social benefits, it is said to be "bigger than <u>Beyoncé</u>" and more accessible.[citation needed]

During the Great Isolation, when many people's daily lives transformed from the post-industrial gig work habits through the quasi-fascist <u>Healthy Life Strategy</u>, an artist now known simply as Cassandra initiated a series of small-group practices known as *The Hologram*, mostly among other precarious artists. In <u>Greek mythology</u>, Cassandra is cursed to utter true prophecies, but never to be believed, leading to the common rhetorical usage of the term to refer to someone issuing unbelievable warnings. In subtle contrast, today the term refers to an accurate prophesy that cannot be believed, but must in any case be adhered to in spite of disbelief to forestall potential calamity.

According to most practitioners and many historians, the historical figure Cassandra was an anxious and self-conscious artist who, early in 2020, released a formula for social participation in "collective health" in the city of <u>London</u>, then the capital of a violent political formation known as a "<u>nation-state</u>" called the <u>United Kingdom</u>. Said to be twitchy and sweaty from having lived a socially complicated and transient life and waging an unsuccessful war against a system of exploitation known as <u>capitalism,</u> lore has it she would say things like "I wonder what a post-individualist feminist economy looks like, and if I can be trusted to imagine it?" (with the voluntary abolition of the <u>Internet</u> some decades later, almost all of Cassandra's written records have been lost). It is believed that she moved to London in the days before the outbreak of the <u>Covid-19 pandemic</u> in 2019. Historians surmise that *The Hologram* was meant to be something artistic and confrontational, in step with the other <u>art</u> of the time. [citation needed]

In a passage widely credited to Cassandra, she describes the way "the Great Isolation granted the canvas needed for many people, who carried the burden of privilege like a pair of golden handcuffs attaching them to a comfortable captivity of reality avoidance, to re-draw their lives and their daily routines." In what many consider to be divine providence, the Great Isolation was the time when *The Hologram* was first being seriously disseminated through workshops and public events on the internet: a now-obsolete addictive network of rudimentary computing machines largely controlled by a violent artificial predatory species known as <u>corporations</u>.

In the years following the event, many <u>psychologists</u> argued that the Great Isolation was an important excuse for people to "discover and strive for what they really wanted, to cancel their plans so they could rest at home alone." [citation needed] It is debated whether the Great Isolation was the cause or the effect of the <u>Great Cutting of the Cord</u>, the beginning of the end of the Internet.

According to the oral history shared by most factions and tendencies that ascribe their lineage to *The Hologram*, at the height of the Great Isolation, most social events and very many meetings related to work and culture began to take place on the Internet including the initial *Hologram* workshops. People from all over the world began to correspond during weekly workshops and meetups led by Cassandra. Thanks to its viral and adaptable nature, within a year of its launch it is estimated that 250,000 people were practicing some version of *The Hologram*. Starting in around 2028, <u>Mondays</u> (a now-obsolete and much-hated period demarcating one full rotation of the earth within an arbitrary cycle or seven such periods developed to expedite the <u>exploitation of labor</u>) were designated the day of <u>Social Holography at Home (Shh)</u> though much folklore suggests that days committed to collective forms of care have been common in human social organization throughout the history of the species. [citation needed] Today, the Shh remains a common cross-cultural name for an extended period when people stay at home and take time to catch up on their contribution to their *Hologram* network.

The success of *The Hologram* is often attributed to the effect of the Covid-19 virus and the social unrest it triggered. In the years following the pandemic the earth lost most of its <u>warlords</u>, both in the sphere known as "government" and the sphere known as "<u>the economy</u>" in a succession of failed rocket launches, where the warlords perished seeking to escape the ecological and social destruction they had unleashed. Most historians agree that sabotage was likely a factor in some if not all explosions. [citation needed] In the vacuum left behind, the practice of *The Hologram* became seamless and ubiquitous on nearly every continent. It started as something quite humble, advertised like a <u>pyramid scheme</u> (a secular and populist capitalist religious practice) and discussed on morning talk shows (a daily capitalist spiritual observance), the earliest written record we have related to *The Hologram*, by an anonymous writer, speaks of it as "women's new work: a way to distribute the compulsory grief associated with the trauma of losing all the world's warlords". [citation needed] But quickly *The Hologram* morphed into a type of <u>party-line</u>, where <u>women</u>, <u>trans</u> people and revolutionaries of all sorts sat on couches, at home, all over the world as they discussed how good they felt about the erasure of power. The practice was used to ensure that health continued as the users of *The Hologram* prepared to defend and protect the new non-hierarchy that had arrived.

Criticisms [edit]

Sometimes referred to as the last laugh of capitalism, no one knows if *The Hologram* is actually as pure as it seems. Elder critics with pre-Great Isolation memory have labeled it a <u>West Coast</u> (referring to the former <u>North America</u> and the land that used to be known as California) <u>Social Practice</u> (an art form labeled by <u>Ted Purves</u> in San Francisco, CA) <u>Cult</u>. It's central organizer, Cassandra, tested positive for internalizing the values and behaviors that she learned from her cultural heritage in the <u>US of A</u> where her death was always the most secure form of long-term stability.

Feminist Economics and the People's Apocalypse

When I was a kid living in an apartment building in the rural areas that would soon consider themselves suburban Chicago, I would sometimes reveal to my mom that I felt poor. One night I told her that I was envious of some kid that had nice clothes and a quiet car. My mom shut off the electric stove and hurled me into her Chevy Cavalier for a drive to the middle-class areas of Grayslake, Illinois, where she took me on a tour of what was and was not behind the cheap windows of the cookie-cutter houses of the "nouveau riche." We visited a new subdivision, which was still mostly a construction site, built directly on top of wetlands and marsh. It was dinnertime or just after in the twenty houses that had been built. We parked in front of a tricked-out house on Lexington Avenue, where each separate room was lit up by a different TV.

My mom pointed and said: "Look at those miserable people!" They have so much money, but they are still alone and suffering! We're miserable too, but they probably don't even talk to each other!"

My mother's (existential?) philosophical performances usually ended in a long drive home, and an apology on behalf of everyone who's ever lived: she never wanted to bring me into a world where everyone was suffering like it's a full-time job. For her, the apocalypse had arrived long ago, and it meant she had to work at terrible jobs where the main protocol was to "stay busy" while wearing loads of makeup. To comfort my sobs she would remind me, "all you have is yourself." This was 1995, the eve of the subprime lending revolution in the Chicagoland area. We would eventually move to Lexington Avenue for a year, claim bankruptcy, and have our own pastel cookie-cutter house foreclosed.

Solidarity: The Known Unknown

A 2007 study by the San Francisco Federal Reserve revealed that the risk of suicide increases when people who earn a lower income live in or close to a wealthier community.[4] "Interpersonal income comparisons" generate scenarios in which one person attempts to keep up with the Joneses, and a poor person's competition with the wealthy defines the value of their life. In this scenario, having less money is a type of death.

As a feminist economist, artist, and financial subject (equipped with the financial literacy training from my mother), I am obsessed with proving that the person who I am supposed to want to be (a ghost person in a nice house with a quiet car) also feels like a miserable failure (alone at night watching TV, as per my childhood education). I'm on a perpetual search for the wretchedness of the supposed "winners" of the game of financial self-management and brutal normativity we are all forced to play. I want to see the soft dark rotten areas in the lives of the wealthy because it makes me feel like less of a loser.

The tendency comes as much out of spite and competition as it does out of love and hope for a collective overturning of everything. By looking into the sour areas in the lives of the wealthy, we might debunk our belief that a wealthy life is the end goal, or that it is even necessarily desirable. Where there is power, money or both, there is also misery and vulnerability because we must debunk our overvaluation of financial wealth (we have no choice). But simply deflating the notion of wealth isn't going to make rich people want to share, or upturn an individuating system of value into a communal one. It's not going to forestall this apocalypse. When you feel powerless and poor it's hard to imagine that anything can be done.

My training as a losing economic subject has led me to a territory called feminist economics, which I want to see as a collective practice and which I can describe in painful detail, but which I cannot yet embody. I associate feminist economics with a kind of collective experience that could reconstitute our idea and experience of risk. Instead of constantly risking everything to survive as individuals economically, we might use our energy to take risks to make collective experiences of steadfast and deep solidarity, wherein success is measured differently—outside of GDP or income bracket.

However, I would characterize this moment as one where my hard-won skills and talents as a self-reliant careerist and a stand-alone survivor might actually work against the practices of a true feminist economist, which would be based on collectively reimagining value. Unfortunately, my expertise as a financial survivor has taught me to put myself first in a defensive mode against the predatory economy that wants to suck me dry, and I don't yet know how to be another way. In the introduction to *Cruel Optimism*, Lauren Berlant admits that the entire book comes through her as a proprioceptive writing—a response that is preconscious, almost muscular—wherein she is a subject who has survived, with scars, the violence of the circumstances she now describes.[5] As an affected subject, I wonder what a post-individualist feminist economy looks like, and if I can be trusted to imagine it?

Economic Violence

> The goal [of the financial industry] is to keep us on the hook until we die, and even beyond the grave …
>
> Andrew Ross, *Creditocracy*[6]

It is important to remind ourselves that a malevolent economic system does not serve life or living. It extracts profit from the people it is meant to serve. Perhaps by identifying financialization as characteristic of the era in which we live, wherein all businesses, services and people are valued by their ability to make money through financial investments instead of from the production of goods, services, social benefits or other forms of value, we are better able to see that malevolence as a system outside of ourselves, and to reject it rather than internalize it.

One byproduct of financialization occurs when social necessary industries like healthcare, housing and education are measured by their ability to generate profit, rather than their function in their intended area of service. We are not financial instruments, and the way that life-supporting infrastructures are motivated by profit is not natural or permanent. Our public infrastructure was not always failing, city budgets did not always rely on police to raise money through fines and healthcare, education and housing were not always too expensive for regular people to afford. Neoliberal economic indoctrination has us believing that we should always be working, progressing and never looking back; we should not have time for non-economic activity, nor for remembering that there are alternatives to this system. In fact, living in a major North American city ensures that we won't be able to do much more than work due to the cost of rent (which increased over two-hundred percent in six years in San Francisco). But the most debilitating by-product of the current economic agenda is that it completely fills our waking hours with work, which is more and more without contract, freelance, a gig, performed alone. If we were to stop producing money, to stop growing our human capital, we would die. Is this true? This set of circumstances teaches us that we can only afford to take care of our individual selves—that we are alone.

This situation is not the same for all of us. While we are all embroiled in this financialized war of class and race, some of us are privileged enough not to feel we have a gun to our heads. There are many forms of direct and indirect violence alive in this financialized moment in the US, the wealthiest society on the planet. My work has largely focused on people (like me) who are slowly drowning but struggling to stay afloat, who encounter a form of wrenching stasis and existential anguish in spite of their relatively privileged position.

Among us, I want to articulate out loud a silent choice we are almost always making. In the midst of police violence, deportation, homelessness and unjust incarceration, we keep paying rent and going to work, pursuing the impossible task of managing our personal risks in a world where the risks are too big and too systemic for us to ever actually succeed. We don't see this as a choice, because it seems impossible to sacrifice our access to our means of survival under financialized capitalism by reaching for an uncharted experience of collectivity, care and mutual aid, abandoning the idea that we can become successful capitalist subjects. How could we let go of what we know are our false and deadly dreams of individual success within this murderous system to construct a yet-unimaginable social world that is organized around people and care?

Even when we make other options transparent, verging on viable, most of us will continue to work to secure a life that is expensive to us (to our health and the planet, socially and financially), but that is familiar and comfortably uncomfortable. In the US, the cost of living is so high that to change our lives, to turn outwards toward the collective, toward protection, feels as if it would cost everything we have and know, even if what we have is mostly debt and what we know is mostly confusion and anxiety. It is a vicious cycle. In our individualized quests to use financial measures to secure our housing, healthcare and education we have learned these lessons of self-sabotage: we are powerless failures that can't do anything right but maybe make money, which will, after all, disappear.

Counter-Professional Surveying Practices for Observing Failure

Perhaps it was because I was always exploring financial crisis in my work that I contracted myself to become my own subject of study: deeply precarious in almost every direction, without stable housing, work, health care, family, culture or community. Americans who experience a medical emergency or death of a loved one are the most likely candidates to file for bankruptcy or lose their homes to foreclosure. In 2015 when my dad died, I missed work and didn't have any money for rent. I understood intellectually that my experience of his death and its repercussions were connected to a broader moment of political, social, and economic apocalypse. Still, the panic that arose from not having money in my bank account was a cry even louder than the loss I experienced. Rolled into my bank account was my tenuous access to my home, my sense of self-worth, my sense of being a failure or a success, my ability to function socially, and the start-up money I needed in order to search for work.

I wanted to learn that I was not alone in my misery. I knew the precarity I experienced was common among other people in my life—though it was invisible. I wanted a way to get people to open up about things they felt too vulnerable to speak of, things that no one would ever even ask about. I was afraid of talking, so I made a survey that could expose how friends deal with the growing lack of conceptual and material stability. I sent it to women and non-binary people I knew. I wanted to learn who else was as uncomfortable in the world as I was, and to hold them closer. This survey was not objective, planned or designed to deliver useful results. It was a cry for help.

We'll look at responses to two questions:

- How often do you run out of money? If you do run out, how do you feel, and what does it cause you to do, internally and externally?
- What forms of economic self-defense do you practice? From scams to jobs, how do you get money?

What the survey reveals is not quantifiable, nor does it provide any economic measurement. It reveals that survival is difficult because underneath a lack of material resources there is not a culture of meaningful participation in shared struggle. When the money is gone, or the work is unavailable, there is nothing safe to fall into. Every failure is a turning point at which the individual has to: pick up and leave town, hide at home, spend day and night hustling or draw tarot cards to give them a vision of a new way to survive. Occasionally, someone takes care of another one, but this is at their own risk—not distributed amongst a community. This mode of individual survival has come to seem so normal, so obvious.

But it's not working. As each person describes their financial problems, inventions and inner struggles they describe how they have been working through the difficulty of material survival in relative isolation, going into economic defense as a lone soldier, or sliding into obscurity with only little sparks of assistance from others. In the cases of those who have not run out of money, it is a rare moment when they see their money as a resource to help others, or a collectively held asset.

I commissioned men advertising their services as spokesmen on Fiverr (a gig-economy website for contracting freelance services) to perform some of the responses to the two most blatantly economic questions in the survey. The decision to deliver the responses in this way was based in my own curiosity—I couldn't imagine what it would be like to see men articulate economic or emotional vulnerability, or openly offer detailed advice, share experiences or to express a desire for solidarity in this way. All in all, my request was rejected by five out of the twenty men that I requested to make testimonials. Their rejection came in one-to-two sentences. They kept it professional by saying that they simply do not perform "this type" of material.

The request I made to the men working on Fiverr acts as a survey with different significance than the original one. If the survey I gave to women and femmes inherently asked, "How are you surviving in this fucked up world, and are you as uncomfortable as I am?" then the survey for men said "Do you have the courage to allow someone else's suffering to enter your body and your online profile?"

Revenge Fantasy

> The body and mind are sensitive and reactive to regimes of oppression—particularly our current regime of neoliberal, white-supremacist, imperial-capitalist, cis-hetero-patriarchy. It is that all of our bodies and minds carry the historical trauma of this, that it is the world itself that is making and keeping us sick.
>
> Johanna Hedva, "Sick Woman Theory"[7]

I want a feminist economics that acknowledges trauma and asks the undercommoners who are tired, hiding, scared or in bed now, who have been stolen from, ignored and violated, what could be offered to repair what has been broken by power and finance, and how. I want it to offer the logic and support to stop the man who insists that the corporate healthcare model is working when, by all measures, exploitation, injustice, inequality and sickness are growing. We need a different way to understand and value our world and culture; we need to center life, not capital; we need to practice real solidarity. This is feminist economics, and the only way to find it will involve collective economic disobedience.

Economic disobedience can take many shapes, and as an individual, you can do it alone as a way to train yourself to overcome the stigma of going against a mainstream ideology. It may help you develop a spinal fortitude to stop believing in and obeying the rules of capitalism. You may stop paying taxes or debts, and you can go off the grid. But any of these actions will result in repercussions that will cost you money, or land you an experience with the (very expensive) criminal justice system, unless you have a network of others supporting you, strategizing with you and leveraging your personal actions into a meaningful political collective social intervention. The free market economy teaches you (and your family unit, if you have one) that you are the only thing you have and the only thing that matters. It is only by overturning that idea in practice that you can really begin to restructure yourself and the economy. But there is almost nothing harder than coming up against the wall: financial capital and all of its laws, social cues and morals. This coming up against the wall—alone, which keeps us from care, from home and from each other—is making us sick.

My revenge fantasy goes like this: someone calls you and asks if you want to be a part of *The Hologram*, the codename for a huge phone-tree shaped network of women, non-binary and trans people and femmes who are in touch, all the time. The shape of the phone tree is actually more like a rhizome, if you could see the conversation network from above. Its path is decentralized and untraceable, undercover in broad daylight because it looks like we're just on the phone, writing letters, sending postcards, Skyping, Google hanging, Facebooking, emailing, FaceTiming, Zooming.

You know, "women's work."

We are asking each other questions about what hurts and where, and taking notes. What are we doing? We are interviewing each other about the conditions of our health, our lives, what it's like to be us. We don't know why we are compelled toward these long and unwieldy conversations, but we can't stop learning about what each others' lives are like. It keeps us alive; it feels like a secret portal to the center of the earth, and back to ourselves. We are asking about the relationships, the mental health histories, the workplace violences, the plants, the nail polish, the family dramas, the addictions, the anxiety, the type of peanut butter and the political aspirations. We are taking notes and we are putting it into encrypted folders. We are following up and asking more questions.

We are Googling radical doctors with lower fees and finding out if a friend really needs the surgery. It feels like the most important work we've ever done, and it is completely invisible—we are here sitting on the couch and no one knows what we are doing unless they are doing it too. For new people, it is difficult and a bit frustrating to understand the degree to which there are no goals besides finding connections, trust and solidarity. The point is that there is a very complex weaving of friendship and collective responsibility, a net that you can't see but you can feel, and it feels strong.

Some people quit their jobs. Not because this is a paid gig, but because when we hear what is happening to those who we've grown to love just across the border, or across some pond, or across a racial divide, we are going to go there and be with them. In this network of phone calls and texts and viral conversations we see that all our crises are connected in varying degrees. And we look back and remember when we thought it was all our fault, that everything was in our head. But it wasn't, and it's not. We account for one another, we hold each other to account and we hold each other, period.

VĀG
ABO
NDS
‾

Appendix I
Art, Debt, Health and Care: An Interview

First published in February 2018

Marc Garrett: Since before the 2008 financial collapse, you have focused on researching and revealing the complex nature of debt through socially engaged art. Your recent work examines health in the age of financialization and works to reveal the connection between the body and capitalism. It turns toward institutions once again to ask how they produce or take away from the health of the artists and workers they "support". This important turn toward health in your work has birthed a series of experiments that actively counter the effects of indebtedness through somatic work, including *The Hologram* project.

The social consequences of indebtedness include the formatting of one's relationship to society as a series of strategies to (competitively) survive economically, alone, to pay the obligations that you have been forced into. It takes so much work to survive and pay that we don't have time to see that no one is thriving. Those who most feel the harsh realities of the continual onslaught of extreme capitalism tend to feel guilty, and/or like a failure.

One of your current art ventures is *The Hologram*, a feminist social health-care project, in which you ask individuals to join and provide accountability, attention, and solidarity as a source of long-term care. Could you elaborate on the context of the project, as well as the practices, and techniques you've developed?

Cassie Thornton: Many studies show that the experience of debt contributes to higher levels of anxiety, depression, and suicide.[8] Debt disables us from getting the care we need and leads us away from recognizing ourselves as part of a cooperative species: it is clear that debt makes us sick.

In my work for the past decade, I have been developing practices that attempt to collectively discover what debt is and how it affects the imagination of all of us: the wealthy, the poor, the indebted, financial workers, babies and anyone in between. Under the banner of "art" I have developed rogue anthropological techniques like debt visualization or auxiliary credit reporting to see how others "see" debt as an object or a space, and how they have been forced to feel like failures in an economy that makes it hard for anyone (especially racialized, indigenous, disabled, gender non-binary or "immigrant") to secure the basic needs (housing, healthcare, food and education) they need to survive, because it is made to enrich the already wealthy and privileged.

After years of watching the pain and denial around debt grow for individuals and entire societies I was so excited to fall into a "social practice project" that has the capacity to discuss and heal

some of this capital-induced sickness through
mending broken trust and finding lost solidarity.
This project is called *The Hologram*.

An Intentional Community in Exile

MG: What kind of people were involved?

CT: The entire time I lived in the Bay Area I
was precarious and indebted. I only survived,
and sometimes thrived, because of the networks
of solidarity and mutual aid I participated in. As
the city gentrified beyond the imagination, I was
forced to leave. I didn't want to let those networks
die. So, at first, the people who were involved were
like me—people really trying to have a stake in a
place that didn't know how to value people over
real estate and capital.

The Hologram project developed when, as I was
leaving the city, I had invited a group of precar-
iously employed, transient activists and artists
to get together in the Bay Area for a week of
working together. We aimed to figure out ways to
share responsibility for our mutual economic and
social needs. On the advice of my friend Debbie
Notkin this project was called the "Intentional
Community in Exile" (the acronym, ICE, is a pun
on the punitive post-9/11 US deportation force
called Immigration and Customs Enforcement,
which became much more pertinent after Donald
Trump's election on an anti-migrant platform
in late 2016). ICE grew out of an opportunity
offered by Heavy Breathing, a "series of experimental, artist-led seminars combining physical

activity with group discussion," to choreograph an event at the Berkeley Art Museum in 2016. They allowed me to go above and beyond my budget to invite a group of eight women together from across the US to experiment with methods of mutual aid: sharing resources, discussing common problems and developing methods for cooperating to co-develop an economic and social infrastructure that would allow us to thrive together, interdependently, even if we were forced to live far apart. What would it mean for our work as activists and artists to feel that we had roots within an intentional community, even if we didn't have the experience of property that makes most people feel at home?

The Hologram was one of many ideas that developed as part of this project. One of the group members, Tara Spalty, founder of Slowpoke Acupuncture (and one of the two acupuncturists you will see at San Francisco protests or homeless encampments), and I fell into the idea of *The Hologram* when combining our knowledge about the solidarity clinics in Greece, our growing indebtedness and lack of medical records and the community acupuncture movement. Then the group brainstormed about what the process would be like to produce a viral network of peer support.

Our Debts, Our Crises

MG: What inspired you to do this project? I'm particularly interested in the Greek influences here and what they mean to you.

CT: For many years I had been doing work about debt, starting from my realization in graduate school that we, students at the California College of the Arts, where tuition cost about $40,000 per year, were actually much more successfully producing debt than art. I hired an actor to pretend to be a student and have a public breakdown on our behalf at my graduate show. I also developed methods of lightly hypnotizing people to get them to actually talk about debt and its impacts on their imagination. And I started an alternative credit rating agency, the idea being to get people's real stories about how living in predatory capitalism puts them in debt, and to train them to collect and share other people's stories in turn. During this time I was also very involved in Strike Debt, a debt abolition activist group that emerged out of Occupy Wall Street.

But my practices of looking at debt became boring to me by 2015. I was becoming more and more clear that individual financial debt was a signal of a larger problem that was not being addressed. The hyper individualism produced by indebtedness allows us to look away from a much bigger deeper story of our collective debts, financial and otherwise. We don't know what to do with these much bigger debts, which include sovereign debts, municipal debts, debts to our ancestors and grandchildren, debts to the planet, debts to those wronged by colonialism and racism and more. We find it so much easier to ignore them.

When visiting austerity-wracked Greece after living in Oakland I noticed that Oakland appeared to have far more homeless people on the street. It made me realize that, while we label some places "in crisis," the same crisis exists elsewhere, ultimately created and manipulated by the same financial oligarchs. Max Haiven and I did a project on how the same hedge funds that profit off of the bankruptcy of the US "commonwealth" territory of Puerto Rico (which many people see as a colony) are flipping houses in gentrifying Oakland and profiting off of the debt of Greece.[9] We're all a part of the same global economic systems. The "crisis" in Greece is also the crisis in Oakland and the crisis in London. For this reason, I have been interested in what we can all learn from activists, organizers and others in crisis zones, who see the conditions without illusions.

Greek Experiments in Radical Health Care

This led me to an interest in the Greek Solidarity Clinic movement that has, since the eurozone crisis, mobilized nurses, doctors, dentists, other health professionals and the public at large to offer autonomous access to basic health care.[10] I went to visit some of these clinics with Tori Abernathy, a radical health researcher. Another project using social technologies inspired by the Greek Solidarity Clinics is called the Accountability Model, orchestrated by the anonymous collective Power Makes Us Sick.[11] The solidarity clinics, of which there are many in cities, neighborhoods and towns across Greece, are run by participant assembly and are very much tied in to radical struggles against austerity. They are staffed by health professionals who donate their time, but also by non-professionals who perform a variety of clinical and administrative roles.

But they have also been a platform for rethinking what health and care might mean, and how they fit together. The most inspiring example for me was in a solidarity clinic in Thessaloniki, the second largest city in Greece. The "Group for a Different Medicine" emerged with the idea that they didn't want to just give away free medicine but to rethink the way that medicine happens beyond conventional models, including specifically things like gender dynamics, unfair treatment based on race and nationality and patient-doctor hierarchies. This group began to work on a project called the Integrative Model which today still operates at the Social Solidarity Clinic of Thessaloniki (SSCT), offering an experimental "healed" version of free medicine.

When new patients came to the clinic for their initial visit, they meet for 90 minutes with a team: a medical doctor, a psychotherapist, and a social worker. The practitioners ask questions like: Who is your mother? What do you eat? Where do you work? Can you afford your rent? Where are the financial hardships in your family?

The team would get a very broad and complex picture of this person and, building on the initial interview, they'd work with that person to make a one-year plan for how they could be supported to access and take care of the things they need to be healthy. I imagine a conversation: "Your job is making you really anxious. What can we do to help you with that? You need surgery. We'll sneak you in. You are lonely. Would you like to be in a social movement?" It was about making a plan that was truly holistic and based around the relationship between health, community and struggles to transform society and the economy from the bottom-up. And when I heard about it, I was, like: obviously!

So *The Hologram* project is an attempt by me and my collaborators in the US and abroad to take inspiration from this model and create a kind of viral network of non-experts who organize into these trio/triage teams to help care for one another in a complex way. The name comes from a conversation I had with Frosso, one of the members of the Group for a Different Medicine, who explained that they wanted to move away from seeing a person as just a "patient," a body or a number and instead see them as a complex, three dimensional social being, to create a kind of hologram of them.

Viral, Holographic, Peer-To-Peer Care

MG: Could you explain how your viral holographic care system works?

CT: At its most basic level three care-givers attend to the wellbeing of one person. Each care-giver represents a different quality of concern. They're not experts or authorities, but people willing to lend attention and to do co-research, to be a scribe or a living record for the person in the center, who we call "the hologram." Our aim is to translate the geographically specific Integrative model of the SSCT into a peer-to-peer project that can be undertaken in a wide variety of places, for a wide variety of crises.

So the beginning of the Hologram process, like that of the SSTC's Integrative Model, is to perform an initial intake where the three care-givers—a triangle—ask the hologram questions which are provided in an online form, about the basic things that help or hurt her social, physical and emotional/mental health. When this (rather extended) process is complete, the hologram and care-givers will meet as a group every season or so to do a general check-in. The goal of this process is to build a social and a physical holistic health record, as well as to continue to grow the triangle of care-givers' understanding of the hologram's integrated physiological, emotional and relational patterns.

Ultimately, over time we hope to build trust and a sense of interdependence so that if the hologram meets a situation where she has to make a big health decision (health always in an expansive sense) about a medical procedure, a job: a move, she will have three people who can support her to see her lived patterns, to help her ask the right questions and to support peer research so that the hologram is not making big decisions alone.

But, in order for the hologram to receive this care without charge and guilt free she needs to know that her care-givers are taken care of as well. So, the hologram has to be proactive in helping all her care-givers to become holograms and find their three care-givers. And so ultimately this expands like a viral network. I think this is one part of the project that acknowledges and makes a practice of the work of feminists and social reproductive theorists: you can't build something new using the labor of people without acknowledging the work of keeping *those* people alive. Reproducing the energy and care we need to overturn capitalism takes a lot of support. Getting support and organization from someone feels so different if you know they, in their turn, are being well taken care of. This is also how we begin to unbuild the hierarchical and authoritarian structures we have become accustomed to: "with empty hands and empty pockets," as Ursula K. Le Guin taught us.[12]

And then the last important structural aspect of *The Hologram* project is the real kicker, and touches on the mystery of what it means to be human outside of capitalism. The real "healing" (if we even want to say it!) comes when the person who is at the center of care turns outward to then care for someone else. So, in addition to the hologram helping her care-givers become holograms. She also becomes one of three care-givers for a different hologram. This is the secret sauce, the goal and the desired by-product of every holographic meeting: to allow people to feel that they are not broken and that their healing is bound up in the health and liberation of others.

The viral structure is built into this system. There is a reversal of the standard way of seeing the doctor-and-patient relationship. In this structure it is essential that we see the work of the hologram as the work of a teacher or explicator, delivering a case that will ultimately allow the care-givers to learn things they didn't previously know. This is the most important, potent and highly-recommended strangers. An "objective" perspective from an outside participant also adds a layer of formality to the project, because unlike a casual gathering of friends an unfamiliar person can add a note of seriousness and focus.

The onboarding process for the hologram and the care-givers includes a set of conversations and a training ritual, which are being developed now. This "training" is a kind of structured personal ritual that allows participants, both the hologram and the care-givers, to witness and adapt their own communication habits so that they feel prepared to participate and set up trust, curiosity and solidarity for the group in the opening intake conversations.

MG: *The Hologram* project was first trialed as part of a cycle of exhibitions called *Sick Time, Sleepy Time, Crip Time*, curated by Taraneh Fazeli which began at the Elizabeth Foundation Project Space in New York City, March 31–May 13, 2017.[13] What have you learnt in more recent undertakings of *The Hologram* project?

CT: Since the original trial in 2017, which lasted for three months, my research has shifted to looking at building skills and answering acute questions that will accumulate to support and build the larger project. Starting in the Spring of 2017, with the support of my inclusion in Taraneh's *Sick Time, Sleepy Time, Crip Time* cycle of exhibitions, I began to offer *The Hologram* project as a workshop where participants could test the implicit communication model. The appearance in these instances has seen me mostly working as a performance artist and rogue architect, creating a situation in a space where people go through a difficult psycho-social and physical experience together.

In the reflective conversations that follow I ask the groups to use the personal pronoun "we" for the entire duration of the conversation. The idea is that one person's experience can be shared by the group. Even as a temporary triangle of care-givers we can take a leap and share their experience with them for a duration of time, allowing a hologram to feel as if their experience is "our" experience. And this feeling that one is not alone in an experience, if carried into other parts of life, has the potential to break a lot of the assumptions and habits that we have inherited from living and adapting to a debt-driven hellscape.

Appendix II

Contextualizing *The Hologram*: Feminist Ethics, Post-Work Commons and Commons in Exile

by Magdalena Jadwiga Härtelova

The Hologram is a project with complex, intertwined roots in participatory art, grassroots activism and radical thought, which, together, present an anarchic garden of interdependent ideas and influences, rather than something that can be presented as if in separate flower pots. Nevertheless ...

Feminist Ethics

As a project attempting to establish a network of vibrant, critically structured channels for interpersonal care, *The Hologram* is a project necessarily and implicitly engaged in ethics. In the Aristotelian tradition, ethics is a call to action, to transformation and to investigation.[14] In our day and age, feminist post-humanities scholar Rosi Braidotti speaks about relational ethics, about "being worthy of our times, the better to act upon them, in both critical and creative manner."[15]

Thornton's project shares post-humanities' action against the patriarchal paragon of "humanity" to which all "others" must try (and fail) to aspire. Together with posthumanism, the interventionist ethics at the heart of *The Hologram* see participating subjects as a collaborative entity, made up of specific embodied actors who are both autonomous and interdependent.[16]

Heralding herself for years under the banner of the Feminist Economics Department, Thornton's work signals its debts to the diversity of feminist thought and its broader insistence that "economics" is not simply a matter of the management of material wealth but of relationships, power and cooperation. *The Hologram*'s foundation in ethics of specificity, difference and embodiedness is the heritage of intersectional feminism, stemming, in Thornton's native United States, from the writings of Kimberlé Crenshaw, Audre Lorde, Gloria Anzaldúa and many, many more who have sought to account for the interwoven nature of multiple systems of power (patriarchy, capitalism, white supremacy, heteronormativity, ableism) as they are experienced in the body.[17] Intersectional feminism, for all its great diversity and debates, shares a commitment to seeing embodied experience, and importantly the shared theorization of that experience, as a key source of knowledge generation. We come to know our world, and to be able to act ethically within it, by working together to understand ourselves in our commonalities and our differences. This is a radical act.

The Hologram's emphasis on specificity and interdependence also resonates with ecofeminist and post-anthropocentric thinkers such as Anna Tsing and Donna J. Haraway. In *Staying with the Trouble*,[18] Harraway demonstrates that our intertwining with other human and "more-than-human" life demands of us a relational ethics and practice, the cultivation of fluid power structures that can "render capable" new, less violent relationships and lead to unexpected outcomes. This kind of deep commitment to the unlikely and the unexpected, to radical re-imagining, animates *The Hologram* and my present attempt to contextualize it.

Post-Work and New, Deeper Time

The Hologram, as a practice and a concept, demands time, commitment and energy. It might be seen as a non-capitalist, non-coercive attempt to reorganize our reproductive labor. Yet for all that, it is also distinctly inspired by post-work imaginaries. Thinkers connected to this socio-economic philosophy, such as Helen Hester and David Frayne, address the ways in which capitalist work, as we know it now, has become an ideology, one that conflates one's job with the value of one's life, one that elevates productivity above wellbeing, one in which we are made to exchange our livelihood for a wage.[19] As a post-work project, *The Hologram* is a kind of revenge on capitalist time, its false scarcity and its perversions of value. In this sense, *The Hologram* has been influenced by the legacy of materialist feminism, emblematized in the famous global "Wages for Housework" campaign of the 1970s, which, as Silvia Federici and Kathi Weeks note, was dedicated not simply to having the value of reproductive labor recognized and remunerated within capitalism, but to abolishing work, capitalist time and the patriarchal separation of productive and reproductive labor completely.[20]

The Hologram's antagonism to capitalist time expresses itself in practices of co-creating a different kind of "slow-time." In her proposal for *The Hologram*, Thornton talks about building a new "world underneath this one," resonating with Tsing's *The Mushroom at the End of the World*, an ode to the life growing through ruins.[21] Einstein's theory of general relativity holds that massive objects with strong gravitational pull influence time itself: time "underneath," near the core of the earth, is slower than on the planet's surface. *The Hologram*, by bringing us into proximity to the weighty core of our shared social life, proposes a slowing of time. In that slowed time we can form an investment in a potential future built on accessible, complex, personalized and interdependent practices of care.

The Hologram's temporal politics and ethics also sensitize us to what is at stake. The "world underneath" of *The Hologram* runs through multiple post-apocalypses. Feminist post-humanism as well as post-work are refusals of the necropolitics of capitalism: the contemporary reality in which the pathological individualism *homo oeconomicus*, rooted in settler colonialism, systemic racism and ableist fascism has led to the social and political power determining who dies and who lives.[22] Contemporary ecofeminism considers how to live a meaningful life on a dying planet, in dialogue with within, against, and beyond the present.[25] After all, *The Hologram*'s key inspiration are the very real Social Solidarity Health Centers in post-financial crisis Greece, a post-apocalyptic, post-time land-scape.[26] Political solidarity movements—whether it is the first of its name, the Polish democratic uprising Solidarnosć,[27] or the anti-austerity Occupy Wall Street—are also reflected in the fluid non-hierarchical structure of *The Hologram*. As was the case in the latter movement, and more generally the case in feminist organizing, in *The Hologram* individual responsibility (for individuals) exists within feedback loops created to question and undermine any push for individuals to take authority.[28] Indeed, Thornton herself was a pro-tagonist in Occupy-aligned actions in the United States, notably Strike Debt, a movement that sought to organize popular resistance to debt, the subject of much of Cassie's early work.[29]

Accordingly, the revolution toward which *The Hologram* strives is not one confined to the dream of able bodies marching triumphantly through the streets in a single event under a great leader. It is, rather, a revolution built on transformed relationships and the activity of commiting time to building "worlds underneath this one." In this, *The Hologram* is informed by lessons of disability activism, notably artist Johanna Hedva's well-cited provocation: "How do you throw a brick through the window of a bank if you can't get out of bed?"[30] Likewise, it attends to some of the challenges around "just checking in" and ableist selfishness posed by artist Sharona Franklin behind the @hot.crip account.[31] Thornton often cites as inspiration the work of critical disability artists Constantina Zavitsanos and Park McArthur, whose work explores debt and (inter)dependency not as flawed expressions but as the very conditions of a shared (post-)humanity.[32]

Taking this kind of radical interdependency as a core, activating value, the project articulates in two streams. On the one hand, it seeks to develop a framework for relationships that accommodate the unique abilities and needs of all participants, informed by curator, educator, critical disability activist and Thornton's long-term collaborator Taraneh Fazeli's observation that, "whether or not we currently identify as sick, we are united by the fact that we all experience fluctuating states of debility throughout our lives."[33] On the other hand, *The Hologram's* focus on interdependency works toward a different, generative understanding of debt, dependence and what it might mean to make an investment, not in financial but in social wealth. As Fred Moten and Stefano Harney explore in *The Undercommons*, whereas a white-supremacist worldview associates debt, poor credit and dependency with weakness and inadequacy, Black community organizing has consistently seen debt as a vehicle for solidarity grounded in the richness of social bonds.[34] Such a transvaluation also resonates with the anti-colonial and anti-capitalist practices of indigenous resurgence, such as those explored by Anishinaabe theorist, artist and activist Leanne Betasamosake Simpson.[35] This influence has grown on Thornton since relocating to Anishinaabe territories in what is currently known as Canada in 2017, where she is actively involved in organizing against settler colonialism with an Indigenous-led feminist street patrol group called Wiindo Debwe Mosewin (Walking Together in Truth).

Thornton also lists among her influences the community acupuncture movement, where patients of this ancient practice are healed by practitioners in a common space, the premise being that their healing is interdependent. Beyond the potent metaphor acupuncture offers for the use of highly precise tiny interventions that have huge transformative impacts on broader systems, community acupuncture also traces its legacies to the Barefoot Doctors of the Chinese Revolution and their inspiration to the Black Panthers and Young Lords, who adapted this medicine to treat the traumas and addictions of white supremacist American capitalism in communities systematically denied health care.

Our Commons in Exile

"Creating worlds underneath" could work as a definition of what has come to be known as social practice or participatory art, sometimes also labeled as relational aesthetics, the shelf in the art world on which *The Hologram* project would likely be placed. When introducing her practice, Thornton declares her ambivalence (or is it affinity?) to the field: "I'm a social practice artist because there is no other word for what I do." The emphasis on creating platforms, spaces, and moments for exchange of attention and knowledge—in other words, using art to establish commons[36]—is a frequent orientation of many socially-engaged art practices. One kindred example is the American anti-racist futurist activism of the *Community Futures Lab*, in which artist and lawyer Rasheeda Phillips and artist and musician Camae Ayewa collected memories with the Sharswood community of Northern Philadelphia in order to re-imagine a local future imperiled by the force of gentrification.[37] Thornton has been deeply influenced by Hamburg-based German theater artist Sibylle Peters who mobilizes the power of collective emotions through transformative storytelling and cooperative research projects to create shared visions for different futures, sometimes as part of the ensemble *geheimagentur* (Secret Agency). Like Thornton, Peters is fascinated by and committed to economic disobedience, creating living, participatory theater pieces with adults and children that invent new currencies and radically re-value people and things to liberate the imagination from the capitalist economy.[38] The notion of rehabituating ourselves to become members of a new society or economy are also key to *Social Presencing Theater*, a project-art genre by Arawana Hayashi, which orchestrates events focused on storytelling and community healing through a combination of performance, therapy and social action research. Thornton has adapted many of these tools in *The Hologram*.[39]

All these projects share with *The Hologram* more than their focus on radical participatory space-making. They are all "art" practices that limit their ties to conventional (art) institutions, seeing them as a means to access resources for social activism and refusing to rely on or contribute to their circuits of cultural capital. The Cuban artist Tania Bruguera calls this "art without art-world permission."[40] *The Hologram*, the *Community Futures Lab* and Sibylle Peters all have roots in traditions of so-called institutional critique, where artists take their own social and economic location as a critical subject. These practices depart from those of an earlier generation, emblematized by the early works of Andrea Fraser, Fred Wilson, or even Mierle Laderman Ukeles (with her focus on maintenance and care) in that they start from the position that much more is at stake than the hypocrisies and complicities of the art world. Indeed, they recognize that such revelations, no matter how critical, can often serve to reproduce that world and its associated economy of money and prestige.

In contrast, the projects put here in the proximity of *The Hologram* draw more from what is labeled as activist art, from its history in political posters, visually symbolic actions and the aesthetics of protests: they focus on gatherings and transformations. They invent institutions and genres of their own in the service of communities in struggle. They are all highly poetic, mixing "practical" steps with allegorical gestures, much as anarchist science-fiction writer Ursula K. Le Guin taught us to move between detailed proposals for social structures and the fantasies of interplanetary travel.[41] Indeed, it would be possible to see all these projects as invested in utopia, if we consider utopia in the radical tradition and its literal Greek meaning as a non-place, a direction.[42] Utopia marks a travel to a destination for the liberated imagination, an invitation to transformation, a portal.[43] *The Hologram*, alongside many examples of anti-capitalist socially engaged art projects, is a collective exercise in radical re-imagination.

But is it Art?

Such re-imagining is a form of cooperative knowledge production. Here, it is based in people's everyday experience of needing, receiving and giving care, yet it shoots toward a different world. The thoughts, practices, and shapes that come together in *The Hologram* project share the value of affective intimacy that enables vibrant knowledge-making based on biographical, experiential and emotional experience. Re-imagining is also a visual act. Part of the reason why social practice art, and with it *The Hologram*, choose to be "art" (rather than, say, "social work" or "education") is because its practitioners are invested in the aesthetic beauty of ideas and relational practices. This commitment to the transformational beauty of concepts and relationships ties *The Hologram* to philosophers of feminist and post-humanist ethics such as Braidotti or Haraway, with whom we began. It also stretches to the futures imagined by activist movements, not in their moments of repose, but in the very nature of their active struggles.

VĀG
ABO
NDS

Notes

1. Helena Smith, "Patients Who Should Live Are Dying," *The Guardian*, January 1, 2017, www.theguardian.com/world/2017/jan/01/patients-dying-greece-public-health-meltdown.

2. Heath Cabot, "The European Refugee Crisis and Humanitarian Citizenship in Greece," *Ethnos* 84.5 (October 20, 2019), 747–71.

3. See Dario Azzellini's film and writing on this occupation:www.azzellini.net/en/films/occupy-resist-produce--viome.

4. Mary C. Daly, Daniel J. Wilson, and Norman J. Johnson, "Relative Status and Well-Being: Evidence from U.S. Suicide Deaths" *Federal Reserve Bank of San Francisco Working Paper* #2007-12, 2007. www.frbsf.org/economic-research/files/wp07-12bk.pdf

5. Lauren Berlant, *Cruel Optimism* (Durham NC and London: Duke University Press, 2011).

6. Andrew Ross, *Creditocracy* (New York: OR Books, 2014).

7. Johanna Hedva, "Sick Woman Theory." *Mask Magazine*, January 29, 2016. www.maskmagazine.com/not-again/struggle/sick-woman-theory

8. William Davies, Johnna Montgomerie, and Sara Wallin, "Financial Melancholia: Mental Health and Indebtedness," London: Political Economy Research Centre at Goldsmiths, University of London, July 4, 2015. www.perc.org.uk/project_posts/financial-melancholia-mental-health-and-indebtedness/.

9. http://universityofthephoenix.com/projects/the-immortal-stranger

10. The CareNotes Collective, ed., *For Health Autonomy: Horizons of Care Beyond Austerity—Reflections from Greece* (Brooklyn, NY: Common Notions, 2020).

11. https://powermakesussick.tumblr.com/

12. Ursula K. Le Guin, *The Dispossessed* (New York: Harper, 1994).

13. www.projectspace-efanyc.org/sick-time/

14. I'm thinking here of Book II in Nicomachean Ethics, among others, where Aristotle demonstrates "virtue" as a state of character in making choices: *Aristotle's Nicomachean Ethics*, transl. by R.C. Bartlett and S.D. Collins (Chicago: University of Chicago Press, 2012), pp. 26–41.

15. Rosi Braidotti, *Posthuman Knowledge* (Cambridge: Polity Press, 2019), p. 3.

16. Ibid., p. 46.

17. For a brief summary about the origins and internal developments of intersectional feminism, see Anna Carasthatis, "The Concept of Intersectionality in Feminist Theory," in: *Philosophy Compass* 9 (5), 2014, pp. 304–14; Kimberlé Crenshaw, "Mapping the Margins: Intersectionality, Identity Politics, and Violence against Women of Color," in: *Stanford Law Review* 43 (6), 1991, pp. 1241–99; Audre Lorde, *Sister Outside: Essays and Speeches* (Berkeley: Crossing Press, 2007); Gloria Anzaldúa, *Borderlands/La Frontera: The New Mestiza* (San Francisco: Aunt Lute Books, 1987).

18. Donna J. Harraway, *Staying with the Trouble: Making Kin in the Chthulucene* (Durham: Duke University Press, 2016).

19. For a summary of much of post-work thought and history, see: Andy Beckett, "Post-work: The Radical Idea of a World without Jobs", *The Guardian*, January 19, 2018 (retrieved 2020-04-27). For consideration of reproductive, care labor within the post-work philosophy, see: Helen Hester and Nick Srnicek, "After Work: What is Left?" [talk, video], kosmopolis.cccb.org/en/edicions/k19/helen-hester-i-nick-

srnicek/ (retrieved 2020-04-27); in anticipation of their forthcoming book, Helen Hester and Nick Srnicek, *After Work: The Politics of Free Time* (London: Verso, 2020); David Frayne, *The Refusal of Work: Re-Thinking Post-Work Theory and Practice* (London: Zed Books, 2015).

20. Silvia Federici, *Revolution at Point Zero: Housework, Reproduction and Feminist Struggle*, 2nd edition (Oakland: PM Press, 2012); Kathi Weeks, *The Problem with Work: Feminism, Marxism, Antiwork Politics and Postwork Imaginaries* (Durham: Duke University Press, 2011).

21. Cassie Thornton, *The Hologram*, pamphlet (Thunder Bay, ReImagining Value Action Lab, 2020), p. 5; Anna Lowenhaupt Tsing, *The Mushroom at the End of the World: On the Possibility of Life in Capitalist Ruins* (Princeton and Oxford: Princeton University Press, 2015).

22. Achille Mbembe, *On the Postcolony* (Berkeley, Los Angeles, London: University of California Press, 2001).

23. Frantz Fanon, *Black Skin, White Masks,* trans. C. Farrington (New York: Grove Books, 1963).

24. adrienne maree brown, *Emergent Strategy: Shaping Change, Changing Worlds* (Chico, CA: AK Press, 2017).

25. Max Haiven and Alex Khasnabish, *The Radical Imagination: Social Movements in the Age of Austerity* (London: Zed Books, 2014).

26. The CareNotes Collective, ed., *For Health Autonomy: Horizons of Care Beyond Austerity—Reflections from Greece* (New York: Common Notions, 2020). Dario Azzellini and Marina Sitrin, *They Can't Represent Us!: Reinventing Democracy from Greece to Occupy* (London and New York: Verso, 2014).

27. In relation to *The Hologram* project, it is especially interesting to look toward the dynamics of self-organizing and found performative powers of the middle european democratic movements, see: Elzbieta Matynia, *Performative Democracy*, 2nd Edition (New York: Routledge, 2016).

28. On the feedback loops used during the Occupy Wall Street movement in-place occupation and their context, see "A World without Power", chapter in *Hyper.Normalisation*, dir. Adam Curtis, London, BBC, 2016.

29. Leigh Clair La Berge, *Wages Against Artwork: Socially Engaged Art and the Decommodification of Labor* (Durham, NC and London: Duke University Press, 2019).

30. Johanna Hedva: "Sick Woman Theory", *Mask Magazine*, Not Again Issue #24, January 2019 (retrieved 2020-04-10).

31. @hot.crip Instagram account, instagram.com/hot.crip/ (retrieved 2020-04-10).

32. Park McArthur and Constantina Zavitsanos, "Other Forms of Conviviality: The Best and Least of Which Is Our Daily Care and the Host of Which Is Our Collaborative Work", in: *Women and performance: A Journal of Feminist Theory*, Vol. 23, Issue 1, 2013, pp. 126-132.

33. Taraneh Fazeli: *Sick Times, Sleepy Time, Crip Time: Against Capitalism's Temporal Bullying* (exhibition catalog) (Omaha, NE: Bemis Center for Contemporary Arts, 2018). Inspired by Eva Feder Kittay terming non-disabled people "temporarily abed" in recognition of the fact that codependency is a reality for all bodies in, Eva Feder Kittay, "Ethics of Care, Dependence, and Disability", *Ratio Juris* #24, 2011, pp. 49–58.

34. Stefano Harney and Fred Moten, *The Undercommons: Fugitive Planning & Back Study* (Wivenho: Minor Compositions, 2013).

35. Leanne Betasamosake Simpson, *As We Have Always Done: Indigenous Freedom Through Radical Resistance* (Minneapolis: University of Minnesota Press, 2017).

36. Silvia Federici, *Re-Enchanting the World: Feminism and the Politics of the Commons* (Oakland, CA: PM Press, 2019).

37. Black Quantum Futurism, www.blackquantumfuturism.com (retrieved 2020-04-10).

38. Max Haiven. *Art after Money, Money after Art: Creative Strategies Against Financialization* (London: Pluto, 2018), pp. 97–100; Paula Hildebrant and Sibylle Peters, "Introduction", in: *Performing Citizenship: Bodies, Agencies, Limitations,* Hildebrandt, Evert, Peters, and col. eds. (London: Palgrave Macmillan, 2019), p. 1. For German speakers, see Martin Elbe and Sibylle Peters, *Die temporäre Organisation. Grundlagen der Kooperation, Gestaltung und Beratung* (Heidelberg und Berlin: Springer Gabler, 2016).

39. Otto Scharmer, *Theory U: Leading from the Future as it Emerges* (San Francisco: Berret-Koehler, 2009).

40. Alex Greenberger, "'Art Without Permission': Tania Bruguera and Dread Scott Discuss Art and Activism at the Brooklyn Museum," *ArtNews*, December 14, 2015, www.artnews.com/2015/12/14/art-without-permission-tania-bruguera-and-dread-scott-discuss-activism-at-the-brooklyn-museum/ (retrieved 2020-04-10).

41. Ursula K. Le Guin, *The Dispossessed* (New York: Harper & Row, 1974).

42. Lyman Tower Sargent, "The Necessity of Utopian Thinking: A Cross-National Perspective," in *Thinking Utopia: Steps into Other Worlds*, J. Rüssen, M. Fehr and T. W. Reiger, eds. (New York: Berghahn Books, 2005), p. 11.

43. Resonating with the walls-portals to other dimensions Cassie Thornton has been creating on gallery and museum walls, see: Magdalena J. Härtelova, ed., *Poznámka k přístupnosti / Accessibility Note* (Prague: Akademie výtvarných umění, 2019), p. 45.

VĀG
ABO
NDS

The Ten of Swords

Pulled and written by Stella Lawless,
The Hologram's Resident Witch

Getting care when we need it most can feel ruinous. Letters from loved ones, past due bills and the junk of credit card "offers" litter the land we need so much to connect with. A plug with no outlet comes out of our soles (souls) and we strive for connection from the depths of our pain. We've been betrayed, wounded and stabbed in the back by systems that make more money the more sick we are. What if all those swords were acupuncture needles? When it gets to the point where we have so much working against us, we have nowhere to go but into rebirth and resurrection. We try too hard to brace against the pain, grimacing and squeezing against how excruciating it is to live in so much disconnection. What happens when we breathe through the pain? When we let go of all the places we're holding? When we roll away from correspondence that adds to our burden and move toward communication and connection that laughs at the absurdity and maybe, just maybe, liberates us all from the isolated aloneness? Mourn in public. The suffering is ending, connection is coming, but we have to begin again. Starting over in a new world where being with discomfort isn't a prerequisite for being alive. I doubt what doesn't exist and strive for it anyway.

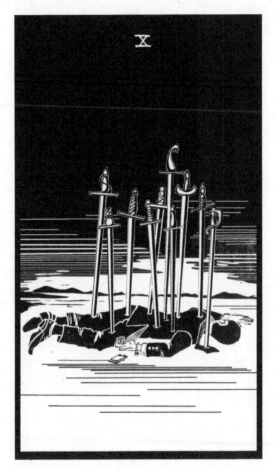

This card, the Ten of Swords, appears as the frontispiece to Max Haiven's *Revenge Capitalism: The Ghosts of Empire, the Demons of Capital, and the Settling of Unpayable Debts*. It was designed by Amanda Priebe who also designed the 'Fool' card that is the frontispiece to this book. As Max's preface to this volume makes clear, our political project and our lives are deeply entangled. When Stella Lawless, my dear friend and resident witch, drew a first card for The Hologram, it was the Ten of Swords and her reading follows. We include it here to signal the close connection between *The Hologram* and *Revenge Capitalism*, projects that are, in a way, two sides of the same card.

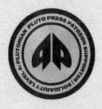

Thanks to our Patreon Subscribers:

Abdul Alkalimat
Andrew Perry

Who have shown their generosity and comradeship in difficult times.